D1083656

RADIATION RISKS
IN
MEDICAL IMAGING

Radiation Risks
in Medical Imaging

JOSEPH P. WHALEN, M.D., F.F.R., R.C.S.
(Honorary. Irel.)

Professor and Chairman
Department of Radiology
Cornell University Medical College,
Radiologist-in-Chief
The New York Hospital-Cornell Medical Center,
Consultant in Radiology
Memorial Sloan Kettering Cancer Center
Rockefeller University

STEPHEN BALTER, Ph. D.

Adjunct Associate Professor of Radiology (Physics)
Cornell University Medical College,
Staff Physicist
Philips Medical Systems, Inc.,
Professional Associate in Radiology (Physics)
The New York Hospital-Cornell Medical Center,
Consultant in Medical Physics
Memorial Sloan Kettering Cancer Center

REF
RC
78
,W5
1984
c.2

®

yb
mp

YEAR BOOK MEDICAL PUBLISHERS, INC.
CHICAGO · LONDON

INDIANA
UNIVERSITY LIBRARY

NORTHWEST

Copyright © 1984 by Year Book Medical Publishers, Inc. All rights reserved. No part of this publication may be reproduced, stored in a retrieval system, or transmitted, in any form or by any means, electronic, mechanical, photocopying, recording, or otherwise, without prior written permission from the publisher. Printed in the United States of America.

Library of Congress Cataloging in Publication Data

Whalen, Joseph P.
    Radiation risks in medical imaging.

    Bibliography: p.
    Includes index.
    1. Diagnosis, Radioscopic—Safety measures.
2. Radiation—Safety measures. 3. Radiation—Dosage—
Standards. I. Balter, Stephen. II. Title. [DNLM:
1. Radiography—Adverse effects. 2. Radionuclude
imaging—Adverse effects. 3. Radiation dosage. WN 200
W552r]
RC78.W5 1983   616.07′57′0289   83-10469
ISBN 0-8151-9254-1

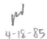

To Liz, Phil, Joey, Mary *and* Charlie

To Shelley, Susan, Kenneth, James, Karen *and* Peter

Acknowledgments

The authors would like to acknowledge the help of the following individuals: Ir. J. den Boer, N. V. Philips, and Bruce Kneeland, M.D., Cornell, for their critical reviews of the draft manuscript; and Joline Cleary, Philips Medical Systems, Inc., and Julia Mala for their assistance in the preparation of the manuscript.

Contents

Tables

ix

Figures

1 / Introduction

Doctor, is that x-ray really necessary? Will it give me cancer, or damage my children? These and similar questions are often asked of practicing physicians as a result of an increasing public awareness of radiation and its risks. This book addresses the needs of the clinician for information regarding patient exposure to, and the potential risks from, the kinds of radiation used for medical imaging. We do not claim that this guidebook is a complete reference to all that is known about the sequelle of irradiation, nor do we claim to have absolute answers to the preceeding questions. We have merely attempted to strike a balance between what is known about the radiation risks associated with diagnostic imaging and other, perhaps more important, risks of life.

Because this is a guidebook, we have included brief discussions of imaging technologies, radiation dosimetry, and radiation biology. Other diagnostic imaging procedures, such as ultrasound and nuclear magnetic resonance (NMR), will be discussed.

We will review the radiation doses delivered to patients undergoing various imaging procedures. These doses are compared to natural background radiation levels and to man-made sources of radiation. At diagnostic imaging levels there is substantial scientific disagreement as to the absolute risks of radiation exposure. Briefly, the controversy is based upon an inability to accurately measure the effects of a single dose of radiation, either as a function of dose level or as a function of the time after the dose is delivered. The difficulty stems from the indistinguishability of either somatic or genetic radiation-induced disease from the naturally occurring variety. Statistical correlations between dose and effect can be made at high dose levels. These statistical methods break down at the levels used for diagnostic imaging. This is due to the small number of radiation-induced lesions relative to the natural incidence of the same disease. The key points in the scientific controversy are reviewed later in this book. The reader will be guided, if he or she desires, through some of the major references dealing with this matter.

There are sections on pregnancy and radiation, fertility effects in the adult and fetal irradiation, and the exposure of both medical and nonmedical radiation workers. Emergency response to radiation accidents is briefly covered.

1

Based on a review of the literature and our experience at The New York Hospital, favorable algorithms will be suggested for the work-up on patients with certain symptoms—sign complexes, or presumed diagnoses. These algorithms will consider the risk of radiation and other risks balanced by the likelihood of obtaining a correct answer. In many cases, multiple "low technology procedures" are replaced by one or a few "high technology procedures" with the bottom line being significant reduction in radiation dose and risk. Obviously, not every clinical situation can be discussed, since that is the content of a textbook of surgery or medicine. The stress of our presentation is on common diagnostic problems, particularly those in which the use of new imaging modalities are important.

It should be also remembered that there are other risks in radiologic examinations, some of which are much more serious than radiation. For example, to mention a few, the incidence of reactions to an IVP[1] is reported as 1 death per 93,320 examinations, cardiac or respiratory arrests, as 1 per 5,760 examinations; and severe hypotension in 1 per 1,952 examinations. Intravenous cholangiography[2] examinations have an even higher incidence of complication, death being recorded in 1 per 5,000 examinations. In performing barium enema examinations, the risks of perforation and embolization exist. One series recorded two perforations in performing 10,000 air contrast examinations. In another report from a large medical center, 13 perforations occurred over a 20-year period.[3] There is a definite risk from the more invasive procedures such as arteriograms, particularly when these diagnostic studies are followed by angioplasty.

It is to be emphasized that since the practicing physician selects the patient for a specific examination to be performed, he or she is responsible for who is irradiated. Since the radiologist is responsible for the conduct of the examination, he or she is responsible for the amount of exposure. In these days of new high technology imaging modalities it is desirable that discussion and consultations take place between the clinician and the radiologist.

Finally, we hope that this book will help the physician to answer his or her patients' questions regarding the uses of radiation in medical imaging.

2 / Sources of Radiation Used in Imaging

THERE ARE FEW BASIC SOURCES that are used to produce the radiations used for the majority of medical imaging. These are x-ray generators, internally administered radionuclides, ultrasonic generators and within the next few years, nuclear magnetic resonance imagers (NMR). In this section, we will briefly review the physical properties of each of these sources and of the radiation that they produce.

DIAGNOSTIC X-RAYS

X-rays are bundles of electromagnetic energy called photons. They can be classified as a portion of the electromagnetic spectrum (Fig 2–1). Because each x-ray photon carries enough energy to ionize matter, x-rays are often called "ionizing radiation." X-ray photons are produced by allowing a current to flow through a high voltage x-ray tube and interact with an internal metal target. The energy imparted to the x-ray photons (a quantity which will ultimately affect the appearance of the finished radiograph) is controlled by adjusting the voltage applied across the x-ray tube. The total number of x-ray photons produced is controlled by adjusting the current flow through the tube and by adjusting the time in which current flow is permitted. It is important to note that x-rays are produced by an x-ray tube only when current is flowing. Therefore, there is no emission of radiation when the x-ray tube is off.

INTERNALLY ADMINISTERED RADIONUCLIDES

Radioactive versions of virtually all of the elements can be manufactured in the laboratory. These radioactive forms (radionuclides) have the same chemical behavior as the nonradioactive forms of the same element. Thus a small amount of the radioactive form of an element can be used to trace the metabolic pathway of that element (such as ^{131}I being used to study iodine pathways) or of a chemically similar element (such as ^{99m}Tc being used to trace phosphorus metabolism).

Radionuclides are unstable and spontaneously decay into other forms by

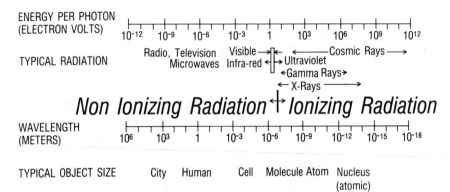

Fig 2–1.—The electromagnetic spectrum.

the emission of particles, photons or both. The radionuclides used for medical imaging emit beta particles (essentially electrons) and gamma rays (the special name for photons emitted by atomic nuclei). The gamma rays emitted by radionuclides as well as those produced by the interaction of a certain type of beta particle (the positron) with tissue are useful for diagnostic imaging.

Since radioactive materials are matter, there are two things that distinguish their radiation properties from diagnostic x-rays when radioactive materials are used: (1) The patient continues to emit radiation until all of the radionuclides have decayed, all the radionuclides have been eliminated from the body, or some combination of both of these processes. (2) A portion of the radioactive material can physically come in contact with another individual, laboratory equipment, bed linens, etc., causing radioactive contamination. The contaminated article physically contains radioactive material and is a source of radiation until the contamination either completes its decay or is physically removed from that article.

One should distinguish between the irradiation of an object and its contamination (Fig 2–2). If an object is irradiated with diagnostic x-rays or gamma rays it will not become a long-term source of radiation. If the same object is contaminated with radioactive material it will act as a source of radiation until the radioactive material is removed by physical means or completes its decay.

DIAGNOSTIC ULTRASOUND

Sound waves are mechanical vibrations in matter. Audible sound consists of those vibrations having frequencies between 20 Hz (Hertz = cycles per second) and 20,000 Hz. The ultrasound used for medical imaging ranges from 1,000,000 Hz to 20,000,000 Hz. The wavelengths of this ultrasound in soft tissue range from 1.5 mm at 1 MHz down to 0.15 mm at 10 MHz.

Ultrasonic energy is absorbed by tissue; the higher the frequency, the more readily it will be absorbed. Unfortunately, high frequencies are needed for good spatial resolution. Therefore, the frequency at which an ultrasonic examination is conducted is determined both by the need to transmit the sound intensity required to form an image and the resolution requirements of the examination.

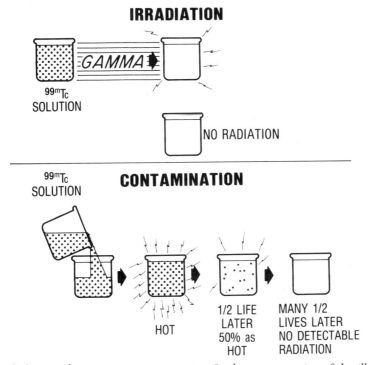

Fig 2–2.—Irradiation is not contamination. In the upper portion of the illustration, the beaker containing pure water can be *irradiated* by bringing it near a source of radiation. In this example, the 99mTc atoms in solution in the left hand beaker are the source of radiation. A portion of the photons emerging from the radiation source and striking the water filled beaker on the right will be deflected (scattered) by the water. When the radiation source is removed, it will no longer irradiate the water. Neither scatter nor any other form of radiation will emerge from the water. In the lower portion of the illustration, the beaker containing pure water is *contaminated* by pouring some of the radionuclide solution into it. Because some of the 99mTc atoms are now physically in the lower beaker, it will act as a source of radiation until those atoms are removed (in this case by radioactive decay). The number of 99mTc atoms remaining in the water beaker will be reduced by 50% for every elapsed half life of the radionuclide (half life = 6 hours for 99mTc).

Medical ultrasound is produced by electrically pulsing a layer of piezo-electric material contained within the ultrasonic transducer (Fig 2–3). The sound pressure pulses are conducted into the patient through the transducer face and a coupling oil. (The oil is required due to the poor conduction properties of air at ultrasonic frequencies.)

When the ultrasound pulse encounters an interface between two dissimilar tissues, it is divided. A portion of the pulse continues distally into the patient. The remaining portion is reflected back toward the transducer. When this reflected pulse reaches the piezoelectric layer in the transducer, its pressure induces an electrical signal. This signal is then processed to form part of the image.

Ultrasonic waves cannot ionize matter. They are therefore classified as nonionizing radiation. (Ultrasound does not belong to the electromagnetic spectrum.) Because ultrasound cannot induce microscopic chemical changes in tissue, one would not expect it to present the same kinds of hazards as ionizing radiation. Ultrasound at diagnostic imaging intensity levels may cause microscopic physical damage. The existence of these effects is a matter of considerable scientific controversy. Ultrasound, if applied with sufficient intensity, can cause macroscopic tissue heating (ultrasonic diathermy) or can mechanically damage tissues by cavitation. Such intensities are well above the levels used for imaging.

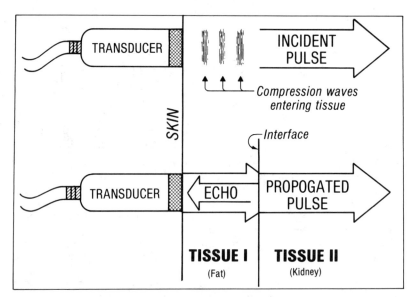

Fig 2–3.—The generation of ultrasonic pulses and pulse echoes in tissue. (See text for explanation).

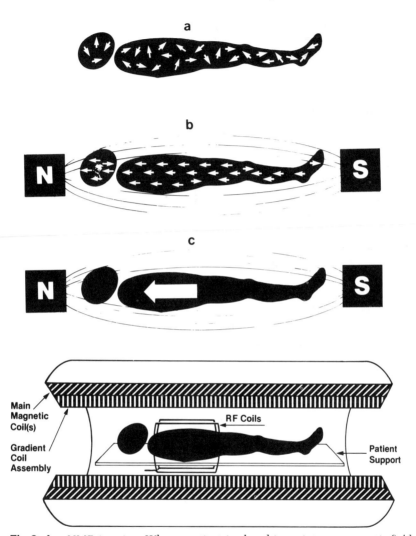

Fig 2–4.—NMR imaging. When a patient is placed in an intense magnetic field, a very small fraction of naturally occurring paramagnetic nuclei **(a)** such as hydrogen, within tissue, are aligned by this field **(b).** This partial alignment produces a small net magnitization in the patient **(c).** This alignment can be probed by subjecting the patient to a pulse of radio frequency (RF) electromagnetic radiation. Information is otained relative to tissue density and composition.

NUCLEAR MAGNETIC RESONANCE

Nuclear magnetic resonance imaging (NMR) is a rapidly evolving modality which uses the electrical and magnetic properties of certain atomic nuclei (such as hydrogen, sodium, and phosphorus) for imaging purposes.[4, 5] When a patient is placed in an intense magnetic field, a very small fraction of naturally-occurring paramagnetic nuclei (such as hydrogen) within tissue are partially aligned by this field (Fig 2–4). This alignment can be probed by subjecting the patient to a pulse of radio frequency (RF) electromagnetic radiation. By properly relating the radio frequency to the magnetic field strength, the nuclei of one kind of atom can be caused to resonate; that is, to absorb energy from the RF pulse and to later emit electromagnetic radiation of the same frequency. If the magnetic field has controlled spatial nonuniformities, there will be a slightly different resonant frequency for each location in the body. One is therefore able to construct an image of the patient by observing which frequencies resonate (where) and how strong each resonance is (how much hydrogen at that location). Other information relating to tissue composition and biochemistry can also be extracted by use of an NMR scan.

It is important to note that NMR imaging does not involve a radioactive decay process. NMR imaging neither requires the injection of radioactive nuclides into the patient nor induces radioactivity into the patient's tissues. Radionuclide imaging and nuclear magnetic resonance imaging are thus two totally different procedures.

3 / Background Material

A LEXICON OF RADIATION UNITS AND TERMINOLOGY is needed to follow the more technical discussions on radiation and its effects. In particular, the reader should note that many of the words used in describing radiation have different connotations from the same words used in the context of pharmacology. We have chosen to use the older system of radiation units in preference to the International System of Units (SI). Conversion tables from conventional to SI units are given in Appendix A.

Exposure

Exposure describes the radiation field, not the interaction of the radiation field with the patient. Exposure is defined and measured by observing the ability of the radiation field to ionize air. The unit of exposure is the *roentgen*. Historically (because on a gram for gram basis air is similar to soft tissue), there is a simple relationship between exposure and dose received by soft tissues. Therefore, in the diagnostic x-ray range, exposure continues to be used as a measure of the radiation energy received by soft tissue.

Dose

Dose describes the energy absorbed by matter from a radiation field. Dose is measured in ergs (energy) absorbed per gram of tissue or other materials. Dose, in a radiologic sense, is similar to the concept of concentration used in pharmacology.

The unit of dose seen in most of the radiologic literature is the rad (1 rad = 100 ergs/gram). Exposing soft tissue to a radiation field of 1 roentgen will result in the tissue receiving a dose of about 1 rad.

Different kinds of ionizing radiation (i.e., high energy neutrons and protons) will cause more biologic damage per rad than will x-rays. Therefore, for some purposes, the dose equivalent (expressed in rems) is used to account for this difference. For the case of diagnostic x-rays interacting with soft tissue, a dose of 1 rad produces a dose equivalent of 1 rem.

When a patient or some other material is exposed to a diagnostic x-ray beam, the absorbed energy is immediately degraded into chemical changes and heat. The patient cannot become radioactive or become a source of x-rays as the result of such an exposure.

9

Dose Distributions

The sizes of the radiation fields typically used for 6iagnostic imaging are smaller than the patient. In addition, diagnostic x-rays are readily attenuated by tissue. Therefore, when a patient is exposed to an initially uniform beam of radiation, the resulting distribution of dose within the patient will be quite complex. Several auxiliary kinds of weighted averages of dose are used to describe the dose distribution in the patient or to the population at large. Figure 3–1 illustrates some of these kinds of doses.

Skin dose is a measure of the dose received by a portion of the patient's skin where the x-ray beam enters the patient. In the diagnostic energy range it therefore represents the maximum dose received by any of the patient's tissues.

Entrance skin exposure (ESE) is a measure of exposure at a location where the patient's skin is presumed to be. ESE is measured using the geometry of the radiographic examination but without a patient (or phantom) present. Because the measurement of ESE is reproducible and because it is related to skin dose, a few government agencies use ESE to regulate diagnostic x-ray exposures.

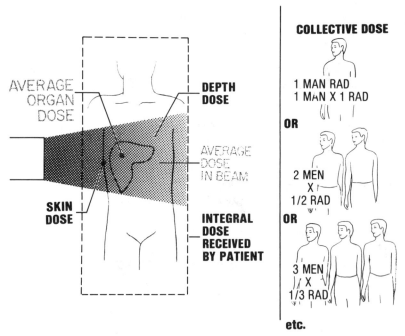

Fig 3–1.—Some of the terms used to describe the spatial deposition of radiation dose. (See text for explanation).

Depth dose is a measure of the percentage of the skin dose found at some depth within the patient. Diagnostic x-rays are readily attenuated by tissue, therefore most tissues within a patient will only receive a small percentage of the skin dose.

Organ dose is a measure of the dose received by a specific organ. For a thin organ, such as the thyroid gland, the dose received by any portion of that organ is approximately the dose received anywhere in that organ (i.e., the organ dose is uniform). For a thick organ, such as the liver, tissue attenuation will cause wide variation in the dose received by different portions of the organ. Therefore, one must take an *average organ dose* as a measure of the dose received by such an organ. Using radiation risk models, one presumes that the risk of irradiating a specific organ is proportional to the average dose received by that organ.

Average dose to the irradiated volume is obtained by taking an average of the dose received by each bit of tissue contained within the geometrically defined x-ray beam. While the concept of this kind of averaging is similar to that of an average organ dose, its utility is less certain. This lessened utility is a consequence of the differing radiosensitivities of different tissues.

The integral dose is a measure of the total amount of energy absorbed from the x-ray beam by a specified mass of tissue. The integral dose received from an x-ray exposure may be defined over an organ, the irradiated volume, or the entire patient. One may assume that the generalized radiation risk from a radiologic procedure is proportional to the integral dose resulting from that procedure. Therefore, techniques that minimize integral dose while improving image quality are to be sought. A good example of such an integral dose minimization technique is x-ray beam collimation.

Collective dose is a measure of the total radiation dose received by a group of people (i.e., the staff of a nuclear medicine laboratory or the population of the United States [population dose]). It is measured in units of man rads (one man rad = 1 man receiving a uniform dose of 1 rad to his entire body). Because radiation injury is known to be both random and infrequent (at low dose levels), one can estimate the radiation risk from an activity by measuring the collective dose resulting from that activity. Therefore, one may not accept a situation that minimizes individual radiation doses (by using many people to perform the work) while increasing the collective dose.

Dose from an x-ray examination: The question of specifying the "*dose received from an x-ray examination*" has no simple answer. As indicated above, there is a complex distribution of *doses* resulting from a single x-ray projection. Most x-ray examinations require more than one projection (i.e., AP and lateral) for their completion. As shown in Figure 3–2, a different

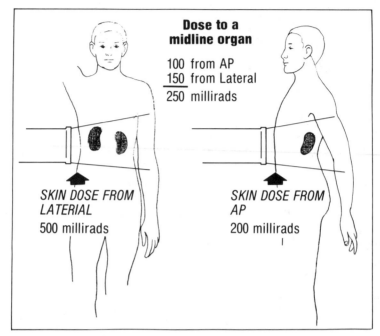

Dose to a midline organ

100 from AP
150 from Lateral
250 millirads

SKIN DOSE FROM LATERAL
500 millirads

SKIN DOSE FROM AP
200 millirads

Fig 3–2.—The "dose from an x-ray examination" cannot be calculated by simple addition or as a simple fraction of the skin dose. For example, different skin doses are required for the two projections due to different patient dimensions in the two directions. In addition, different portions of the patient's skin are irradiated for different projections. Also the distance between the skin and an organ will vary with the radiographic projection. Due to an exponential fall off of depth dose as a function of distance in the patient, the effective depth dose will vary with the projection.

portion of the patient's skin is irradiated for each projection. In addition, the organ dose for a particular organ resulting from each projection will be a function of both the technical factors and of the patient's anatomy. The total dose cannot be uniquely specified by adding up all of the skin doses. The generalized radiation risk may be estimated grossly by adding the integral doses. A detailed dose assessment requires individualized calculation of both dose and tissue distributions.

Genetically significant dose (GSD) is the radiation dose received by the active gene pool of the population. GSD is calculated by multiplying the gonadal dose by a weighting factor. This weighting factor is the expected number of future children of the irradiated individual. Irradiation of individuals who are beyond their reproductive years will not contribute to the GSD.

Radionuclides

The activity of a sample of a radionuclide is a measure of the number of radioactive transformations occurring in that sample in one second. The unit of activity is the Curie (1 Ci = 3.7×10^{10} transformations per second, approximately the activity of one gram of radium). Typical doses (administered quantities) used for radionuclide imaging range from a few microcuries to about 20 millicuries. The exact amount of activity administered in any single study will depend upon the nature of the study, the physical characteristics of the radionuclide and the biochemical behavior of the administered radiochemical. The radiation dose received by the patient, and by specific organs within the patient, will also be a complex function of the preceding factors.

In particular, one should note that the nonuniform distribution of a radionuclide that is essential to imaging results in a nonuniform dose distribution within the patient (Fig 3–3).

Ultrasound

The output of a medical ultrasonic transducer is usually specified in terms of power density (milliwatts per square centimeter). Ultrasonic imaging is usually performed by putting brief pulses of sound energy into the patient and waiting between pulses for the echoes to return. Typical imaging units have a transmitter duty cycle (percent of time the transducer is emitting sound waves) of about 0.1 percent. One may therefore specify either the peak power (power emitted while the transducer is actually transmitting) or the average power (averaged over one second).

In addition, all portions of the transducer do not emit ultrasound uniformly. One therefore can choose to specify either the spatial peak power (maximum from anywhere on the transducer) or spatial average power (averaged over the entire transducer face).

Because ultrasound power meters, historically, were capable of measuring with great spatial resolution and poor temporal resolution, the output of diagnostic ultrasound equipment is usually specified in the hybrid unit SPTA. This unit stands for *spatial peak temporal average* and is quite descriptive of the measuring process. It simply represents the time averaged output of the most highly emitting portion of the transducer.

Nuclear Magnetic Resonance

During the process of NMR imaging the patient is exposed to three separate kinds of electromagnetic fields. These are:

The *main magnetic field* (used to align the atomic nuclei). Typically the strength of the main magnet is 1,000 to 15,000 gauss. This field is maintained during the imaging procedure and is often called the static field. The strength of the earth's magnetic field is approximately one gauss. The

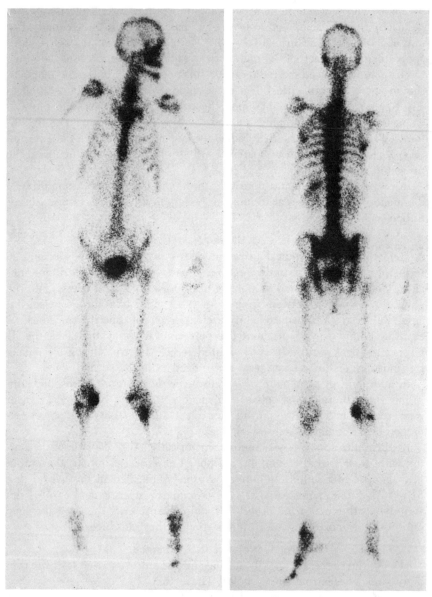

Fig 3–3.—Nuclear medicine—radionuclide scan. ^{99m}Tc labelled bone scan demonstrating a nonuniform distribution of the radionuclides.

magnetic field strength may be specified in terms of the SI unit, the tesla (1 tesla = 10,000 gauss).

Gradient magnetic fields (used to define the imaging space). These auxiliary fields are rapidly switched during the imaging sequence for the purpose of spatial localization of the resonance. The switching rates of the gradient fields are defined in units of gauss per second (tesla per second) at any location within the patient.

Radio frequency fields (used to cause the atomic nuclei to resonate). Typically the RF pulses irradiate the patient with a total average power of 50 to 500 watts. The spatial distribution of the RF heating may be of concern as well as the total heating effect of the RF field. This RF heating may be compared with the patient's basal metabolic rate of 100 watts.

BACKGROUND RADIATION

Life has evolved with a certain amount of external and internal background radiation as a natural portion of the environment. This background radiation has been a part of the world since the beginning of time and therefore cannot be considered as an environmental pollutant peculiar to the twentieth century. Under ordinary circumstances, the amounts of naturally-occurring background radiation, and the variation in the amount of background radiation from place to place, are not considered important by many people. The average U.S. population dose increment from diagnostic imaging is approximately the average U.S. external background dose.

Consider an average individual living in a typical environment at sea level. This individual will be exposed to several sources of external and internal natural background radiation as well as several sources of manmade radiation. If the natural background radiation is much more intense than the man-made contribution, we can logically assume that most of the effects of radiation on this individual are due to natural causes. (A discussion of the distinctions between partial and whole body irradiations appears later in this chapter).

At sea level about half of the external natural background radiation level is due to cosmic radiation. Cosmic radiation consists of high energy photons as well as various species of atomic and subatomic particles.

Low levels of this cosmic radiation are present everywhere in the universe. Some of this cosmic radiation penetrates through the shielding effects of the earth's atmosphere and thereby contributes to the background radiation experienced by an individual. The earth's atmosphere actually acts as a reasonably efficient absorber of the cosmic radiation coming in from outer space. It can be demonstrated easily that the higher one goes above sea level, the greater the intensity of ambient cosmic radiation. Two locations differing in altitude by a mile have a cosmic ray intensity which differs by a factor of two. An individual living on the side of a mountain will be living with twice the environmental cosmic ray intensity as will an individual living at sea level. The increase in cosmic ray intensity with increasing altitude can also be observed easily during the flight of high altitude commercial jet liners.

The second main contribution to external environmental background radiation is that due to the naturally-occurring radioactive material present in the ground, water and air that surround us. Most of this terrestrial background radiation comes from a minute uranium content present in most rock. An individual living in a normal sort of house in the New York area would receive about half of his or her background radiation from this source. Since the uranium content of different rocks will vary widely, the terrestrial contribution to background radiation will vary depending upon location. Indeed, the amount of terrestrial background radiation is influenced by the way in which we choose to live. A person living in a brick house, for example, will be exposed to a slightly higher level of terrestrial radiation coming from the uranium content in the brick and cement of which the house is constructed. If the house is well sealed to prevent heat losses, there will be a further build up of both external and internal background radiation due to an accumulation of radon (a decay product of uranium) in the house. This radon concentration has recently become a matter of discussion among public health authorities. However, an individual living in a wood frame house would be exposed to a slightly higher level of cosmic radiation since wood is a less efficient absorber of cosmic radiation than is brick and stone. The ability to measure these differences is a tribute to the technology of sensitive measuring techniques and instruments.

Some of the larger values of terrestrial radiation are found in a portion of the Amazon River basin in Brazil and in an area near Madras in India. The natural environmental radiation levels in both of these locations are above 500 millirads per year. (The worldwide average natural external background level is 100 millirads per year.) There have been extensive studies on people living in these areas looking for evidences of radiation effects attributable to these high background levels. There have been no demonstrated differences in longevity, disease prevalence, genetic abnormality, mental or physical abilities in these populations when compared to similar populations living in lower background radiation areas.

A third natural contribution to background radiation comes from the naturally-occurring radioactive materials present in all living things. These radionuclides are naturally present in food, air, and water. Small quantities of tritium, potassium-40 and carbon-14 are present in every living organism; for example, in a tree. They are acquired by the organism by inhalation or as part of the food chain. The nonuniform distribution of these natural quantities of naturally-occurring radionuclides (as well as artifically enhanced quantities of natural or man-made radionuclides) within the body should be noted. Such distributions lead to the presence of areas of high local concentration of the radionuclide or "hot spots." Local dose rates in the vicinity of these "hot spots" are of concern. However, a detailed discussion of this problem is beyond the scope of this publication.

RELATIVE RADIATION LEVELS

A preliminary scale of the radiation levels received by a patient undergoing diagnostic imaging is presented in Table 3–1. Relative dose levels are indicated in terms of numbers of "chest x-rays." This presentation is for didactic purposes only; there is no implication that this scale has any simple correlation with relative radiation effects. Nevertheless, radiation levels are scaled in this way for two reasons: The first reason follows from the usual conservative assumption that radiation risk is proportional to radiation dose. Since a majority of x-ray examinations are chest exams, such a qualitative guide may be useful to the clinician. Many competent scientists think that any simple comparison between partial body doses and total body doses is invalid. Others accept such comparisons as reasonable semiquantitative estimates of relative radiation risks. The second reason is, by

TABLE 3–1.—Gross Comparison of Relative
Radiation Levels*

	SCALED RELATIVE DOSE†
Natural background	50–100 chest examinations/year
Diagnostic radiology	0.1–500 chest examinations/study‡
Nuclear imaging	50–1,000 chest examinations/study¶
Start of acute radiation syndrome	30,000 chest examinations in *one* day
Lethal dose (LD50$_{30}$)	300,000 chest examinations in *one* day
Radiation therapy (small volumes of tissue)	100,000–1,000,000 chest examinations in a few weeks
Ultrasound	This scale does not apply
NMR	This scale does not apply

*Due to differential tissue distributions and sensitivities, such estimates are intended to be rough comparisons (50–100 chest examinations will have different biologic effects from that resulting from 100–200 mrads of natural background).

†1 PA chest examination = 5 millirad average tissue dose in thorax which corresponds to a whole body equivalent dose of 2 millirads.

‡Dependent on examination types and techniques.

¶Does not properly account for doses received in those tissues in which the radionuclide concentrates.

analogy, between radiation and pharmaceuticals. In particular, the ratio between the useful dose of radiation and the acute lethal dose is much greater than that possessed by most pharmaceuticals.

Again, before proceeding into a detailed discussion of radiation levels and effects, we have presented relative radiation levels of various sources expressed in proportion to the whole body equivalent of a typical PA chest radiograph. We do this knowing that due to differential tissue distribution and sensitivities such a comparison is a gross approximation to reality (i.e., 50 to 100 chest examinations will have different biologic effects than 100 to 200 mrad a year background radiation). In an effort to calculate inhomogeneity effects, the International Commission on Radiological Protection[6] has adopted a formal system of dose weighting for nonuniform irradiation. The weighted dose equivalent limits are intended to give equal stochastic risk whether the irradiation is homogeneous or inhomogeneous (averaged over the whole body). Such a calculation is useful for developing radiation protection guidelines for occupational exposures. Its extension to diagnostic imaging is not well established and will not be considered in this monograph.

OTHER RADIATION SOURCES

The population is exposed to a wide variety of radionuclides and other sources of ionizing radiation.[7] A partial list includes such obvious items as nuclear reactors, radioactive wastes and ionization-type smoke detectors. It also includes less obvious items as self-luminous watch and clock faces and stray radiation from television receivers. Even less obvious items should be included such as some construction materials, artificial tooth porcelains and optical glass. Smoking concentrates the naturally-occurring radionuclides in tobacco onto the smoker's bronchial epithelium. Such a listing can easily be expanded to fill a book. We will therefore briefly review a few principals rather than try to be exhaustive in our catalog and description of these miscellaneous sources.

In general, whole body exposures resulting from these sources are of very low-level. The generalized risks from such exposures are much lower than the individual benefits gained by permitting such uses of radiation. There are, however, areas of real concern relative to these public exposures to radiation. The most obvious concern is the "what if" scenarios relative to nuclear accidents. Another obvious area of improvement is the substitution of less dangerous or nonradioactive materials where possible. Such substitutions include the replacement of radium by tritium in watch dials, the elimination of uranium in dental porcelain, etc.

The more or less voluntary concentration of radionuclides, particularly alpha particle emitters, has become an area of concern to the public health authorities in the past few years. Two origins for such concentrations are smoking (as mentioned above, this leads to the entrapment of radionuclides in the smoker's lung) and thermal sealing of buildings (leading to an increase in radon concentration in the air due to the decreased air circulation, followed by a build-up of radon daughter radionuclides in the lung). These concentrations of alpha emitters produce localized areas with very high dose equivalents (hot spots). Some authorities believe that the local irradiation resulting from the hot spots is the cause of a significant fraction of lung cancers.

To conclude this section, exposures of the population to a broad range of environmental radiations are known and the dosimetric consequences of such exposures can be calculated. Even though the radiation levels are low, for many years efforts have been underway which are directed toward the reduction of unnecessary irradiation. Some voluntary exposures may indeed have significant health consequences. Dealing with these exposures is a real and unsolved public health problem.

RISK

The doses resulting from the range of radiologic imaging procedures will be presented in later sections of this monograph. With the possible exception of radiation-induced congenital abnormalities (resulting from an in utero high level exposure of a viable fetus), the radiation risk from diagnostic imaging is said to be stochastic. A stochastic effect is one where *probability of occurrence* in an exposed population (rather than its severity in an affected individual) is proportional to the radiation dose received by the total population. One should carefully consider the implications of nonstochastic and stochastic risks. We can illustrate the point by considering the benefits of investing one hundred dollars. One can invest nonstochastically by putting the money into an insured savings account. In this case, one is certain to have a return of one's principal and interest. One can also "invest" the money stochastically by buying a ticket in the Irish Sweepstakes. In this case, there is only a small probability of gaining any money back. The lucky few whose tickets are drawn for the final race are certain to have some return, but even for these few the amount of their winnings is determined by an outside event (the horse race).

In the case of a stochastic risk (at diagnostic imaging levels in particular) the odds are heavily in one's favor that a given dose of radiation will cause no noticeable injury. An unlucky few will sustain a radiation injury. The severity of expression of this injury will depend upon nonradiologic events (treatment, death from an unrelated disease before the radiation injury is manifest, biorepair, etc.).

LEAGUE OF WOMEN VOTERS	COLLEGE STUDENTS	BUSINESS AND PROFESSIONAL CLUB MEMBERS
NUCLEAR POWER	NUCLEAR POWER	HANDGUNS
MOTOR VEHICLES	HANDGUNS	MOTORCYCLES
HANDGUNS	SMOKING	MOTOR VEHICLES
SMOKING	PESTICIDES	SMOKING
MOTORCYCLES	MOTOR VEHICLES	ALCOHOLIC BEVERAGES
ALCOHOLIC BEVERAGES	MOTORCYCLES	FIRE FIGHTING
GENERAL AVIATION	ALCOHOLIC BEVERAGES	POLICE WORK
POLICE WORK	POLICE WORK	NUCLEAR POWER
PESTICIDES	CONTRACEPTIVES	SURGERY
SURGERY	FIRE FIGHTING	HUNTING
FIRE FIGHTING	SURGERY	GENERAL AVIATION
LARGE CONSTRUCTION	FOOD PRESERVATIVES	MOUNTAIN CLIMBING
HUNTING	SPRAY CANS	LARGE CONSTRUCTION
SPRAY CANS	LARGE CONSTRUCTION	BICYCLES
MOUNTAIN CLIMBING	GENERAL AVIATION	PESTICIDES
BICYCLES	COMMERCIAL AVIATION	SKIING
COMMERCIAL AVIATION	X RAYS	SWIMMING
ELECTRIC POWER	HUNTING	COMMERCIAL AVIATION
SWIMMING	ELECTRIC POWER	ELECTRIC POWER
CONTRACEPTIVES	FOOD COLORING	RAILROADS
SKIING	PRESCRIPTION ANTIBIOTICS	SCHOLASTIC FOOTBALL
X RAYS	MOUNTAIN CLIMBING	CONTRACEPTIVES
SCHOLASTIC FOOTBALL	RAILROADS	SPRAY CANS
RAILROADS	BICYCLES	X RAYS
FOOD PRESERVATIVES	SKIING	POWER MOWERS
FOOD COLORING	SCHOLASTIC FOOTBALL	PRESCRIPTION ANTIBIOTICS
POWER MOWERS	HOME APPLIANCES	HOME APPLIANCES
PRESCRIPTION ANTIBIOTICS	POWER MOWERS	FOOD PRESERVATIVES
HOME APPLIANCES	VACCINATIONS	VACCINATIONS
VACCINATIONS	SWIMMING	FOOD COLORING

Fig 3–4.—Perception of Risks. Ranking given by League of Women Voters,

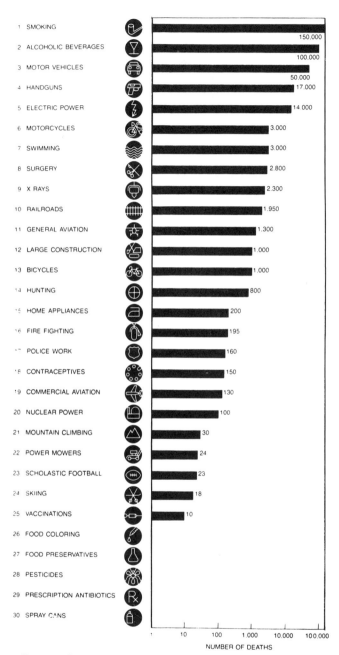

		Number of Deaths
1	SMOKING	150.000
2	ALCOHOLIC BEVERAGES	100.000
3	MOTOR VEHICLES	50.000
4	HANDGUNS	17.000
5	ELECTRIC POWER	14.000
6	MOTORCYCLES	3.000
7	SWIMMING	3.000
8	SURGERY	2.800
9	X RAYS	2.300
10	RAILROADS	1.950
11	GENERAL AVIATION	1.300
12	LARGE CONSTRUCTION	1.000
13	BICYCLES	1.000
14	HUNTING	800
15	HOME APPLIANCES	200
16	FIRE FIGHTING	195
17	POLICE WORK	160
18	CONTRACEPTIVES	150
19	COMMERCIAL AVIATION	130
20	NUCLEAR POWER	100
21	MOUNTAIN CLIMBING	30
22	POWER MOWERS	24
23	SCHOLASTIC FOOTBALL	23
24	SKIING	18
25	VACCINATIONS	10
26	FOOD COLORING	
27	FOOD PRESERVATIVES	
28	PESTICIDES	
29	PRESCRIPTION ANTIBIOTICS	
30	SPRAY CANS	

1   10   100   1.000   10.000   100.000

NUMBER OF DEATHS

college students, and business and professional club members compared to actual number of deaths.

The risk of radiogenic injury from a diagnostic x-ray examination will depend upon the body part being irradiated, the technical parameters of the examination and the size of the patient. As a very crude figure, the authors estimate that the risk of cancer induction from a diagnostic examination is in the range from 1 case per 10,000 exams to 1 case per 1,000,000 examinations. The natural risk of cancer induction is 1 in 6. (A sample calculation appears in Chapter 7.)

In the context of risk, exposure to diagnostic x-rays is conceptually equivalent to a small risk of an accident's occurring during the procedure. The more often a patient is irradiated, however, the more often the patient is exposed to the risk of an accident. Even though the vast majority of individual diagnostic x-ray examinations (over 99.99%) will cause no radiogenic

TABLE 3–2.—Estimated Loss of Life
Expectancy Due to Various Causes*

LIFESTYLE	ESTIMATED LOSS IN DAYS
Being unmarried—male	3,500.
Cigarette smoking—male	2,250.
Being unmarried—female	1,600.
Cigarette smoking—female	800.
Dangerous job	300.
Motor vehicle accidents	207.
Alcohol (U.S. average)	130.
Accidents at home	95.
Average job	74.
Radiation job	40.
Accidents to pedestrians	37.
Safest job	30.
Natural radiation	8.
Medical x-rays	6.

INDIVIDUAL ACTION	ESTIMATED LOSS IN MINUTES
Buying a small car	7,000.
Coast to coast drive	1,000.
Coast to coast flight	100.
Smoking a cigarette	10.
Calorie-rich dessert	50.
Non-diet soft drink	15.
Diet soft drink	0.15
Crossing a street	0.4
Extra driving	0.4/mile
Not fastening seat belt	0.1/mile
1 mrem of radiation†	1.5

*Adapted from Cohen and Lee.[8] Reproduced from *Health Physics*, 36:707, 1979. Used by permission of the Health Physics Society.
†See Appendix A for definitions of radiation units (1 chest x-ray ~ 5 mrem to the thorax).

injury, the exposure of whole populations to screening examinations entails some risk to the population as a whole.

Another way of assaying the hazards of radiation is to compare the risks of irradiation against the risks associated with some of life's other hazards. Cohen and Lee[8] have recently published a comprehensive "Catalog of Risks." Table 3–2 is abstracted from their publication. This paper and the values abstracted from it in our table have provoked a great deal of discussion among epidemiologists. In particular, there is little information relating to the statistical uncertainties of the numerical values given in their tables. Also, Cohen and Lee[8] chose to present their estimated risk data in terms of actuarial life shortening (averaged over the entire U.S. population). While this process permits a relatively simply perceived comparison between differing small risks, it confounds the distinction between voluntary and involuntary risks. The reader must therefore use this data as a general guideline. No precision is implied by the authors of this monograph in reprinting Cohen and Lee's data. Many relationships can be observed in Table 3–2. In particular, the risk of a chest x-ray (5 millirads average dose to the thorax) can be grossly compared to the risk of drinking a cola or smoking a cigarette.

Public and professional perceptions of the benefits and risks of any given activity will lead to its acceptance or rejection. Often these perceptions will differ markedly from the actual risks. The ultimate decision as to the acceptability of any risk, including radiation, is one in which society as a whole should be represented. The public appears to overestimate the risks of radiation.[9, 10] Fischoff[11] has studied the public perception of a wide variety of risks by members of three different groups (League of Women Voters, College Students, Business and Professional Club Members). The results of this study are shown in Figure 3–4. It is therefore no surprise to find great public pressures directed toward reducing the uses of radiation.

There is a need to communicate a balanced picture of radiation risks and benefits to the public. It must be hoped that such a full disclosure will ultimately lead to a public policy which is more or less in balance with the actual risks and benefits of radiation use.

The psychological stresses associated with public perception of radiation risks from nuclear power has recently become a field of study in its own right. Indeed, the U.S. Nuclear Regulatory Commission has been petitioned to consider the psychological aspects of radiation exposure and potential radiation accidents when reaching their decisions.

4 / Imaging Procedures and Doses

RADIOGRAPHIC EXAMINATION

A RADIOGRAPHIC IMAGE IS FORMED by allowing an x-ray beam to impinge upon a patient. X-rays are differentially attenuated due to differences in tissue thickness, density and composition. The differential attenuation modulates the x-ray beam which leaves the patient and goes on to produce the final radiographic image. The modulation is partially controlled by adjusting the voltage applied to the x-ray tube. In general, the lower the voltage the more contrast in the radiograph and the higher the patient *dose*. Radiologic technique seeks to balance the need for contrast and other imaging parameters against the desire to minimize patient dose.

The modulated x-ray beam is intercepted by the radiographic cassette. Intensifying screens, which are found within the cassette and which consist of layers of fluorescent crystals, absorb a large fraction of the modulated x-ray beam, fluoresce, and thereby convert the x-ray image into a light image. This light image exposes a sheet of film, which is subsequently processed into a finished radiograph.

Enough x-rays must penetrate the patient so as to produce both adequate film blackening and acceptable image granularity. The quantity of radiation incident on the patient will therefore be dependent both on the nature of the x-ray beam and upon the attenuation by the patient. Thick or dense body parts will require more radiation *dose* than thin parts. The patient's skin dose is minimized by preferentially removing the nonpenetrating portion of the x-ray beam (i.e., the low energy portion) by means of an aluminum plate, called a filter, between the x-ray tube and the patient. (Some special studies use materials other than aluminum as filters.)

The integral dose received by the patient can be minimized by collimating the x-ray beam to the area of interest. In this manner, tissues not required to be imaged for diagnostic purposes need not be irradiated.

There have been many studies of the radiation *dose* associated with radiologic procedures in the past decades. The most comprehensive United States study was the X-Ray Exposure Study-1970 (XES-70) conducted by the U.S. Bureau of Radiological Health (BRH). (BRH has been recently incorporated into the newly formed National Center for Devices and Ra-

24

diological Health. In a historical sense, we shall still refer to this component of NCDRH as BRH.) Data was collected by the National Center for Health Statistics.[12] While BRH has conducted limited studies in the past decade, such as the Nationwide Evaluation of X-Ray Trends[13] (NEXT) series, the XES-70 data represents the best presently available national information. Surveys such as NEXT are conducted on a limited basis in terms of geographic region (only 17 states were included in the 1980 survey) and in terms of the numbers of examinations studied.

Data obtained from XES-70[14] and NEXT-80[15] for a few representative radiographic studies are given in Table 4–1. Detailed comparisons between NEXT-80 and XES-70 are hampered by a difference in dose measurement techniques and major differences in the calculation model used to derive organ doses from skin doses. The comparison presented here is useful to estimate gross trends in radiation dose over the intervening decade.

Mammography

Mammography is a special example of a radiographic examination. Mammographic examinations require relatively high *doses* because of their exacting image quality requirements. In addition, the female breast is more radiosensitive than most tissues.

Two principal examination techniques are presently in use: xerographic and film-screen. The xerographic technique uses a tungsten target x-ray tube operated at 40 to 50 kVp together with an aluminum filter and a xerographic image receptor. The film-screen technique uses a molybdenum target x-ray tube operated at 25 to 40 kVp together with a molybdenum filter and an intensifying screen-film combination as the image receptor.

These two techniques produce markedly different images, the relative merits of which will not be debated in this monograph. Fundamental physical differences in the x-ray beams give rise to significant differences in the dose distributions within the breast.[16] In this case, knowledge of only the skin dose, and not the technical factors, can lead to major errors in estimating the average breast dose. One cannot, therefore, assume equal organ dose and, therefore, risk, for film and xeromammograms even though the skin dose might be equal for each projection in both studies.

FLUOROSCOPIC EXAMINATION

An x-ray image used for fluoroscopy is produced in the same general manner as the radiographic image. The conversion of the modulated x-ray beam into an image differs from the radiographic case. Moreover, fluoroscopy has changed radically in the last quarter century due to the introduction of the x-ray image intensifier.

TABLE 4–1.—REPORTED DOSES FROM TYPICAL DIAGNOSTIC X-RAY EXAMS
(U.S. PUBLIC HEALTH SERVICE)

Survey:		NEXT-1980			XES-70	
Quantity:		INTEGRAL SURFACE EXPOSURE[c]	MEAN ENTRANCE SKIN EXPOSURE (NO BACKSCATTER)[d]	MEAN ACTIVE[a] MARROW DOSE	MEAN ENTRANCE SKIN EXPOSURE (WITH BACKSCATTER)[d]	MEAN ACTIVE[a] MARROW DOSE
Unit:		Roentgens x cm^2	milliRoentgens	millirads	milliRoentgens	millirads
Projection						
Chest PA	$\bar{x}$[b]	27	22	2	36	5
	s	2	3	—	2	—
Skull LAT	$\bar{x}$	103	196	6	420	17
	s	13	26	1	27	1
Abdomen AP	$\bar{x}$	444	581	20	951	92
	s	30	49	2	52	6
Cervical spine	$\bar{x}$	70	162	2	514	19
	s	11	23	2	83	3
Thoracic spine	$\bar{x}$	265	402	12	1,050	120
	s	39	33	1	112	14
Lumbosacral	$\bar{x}$	454	641	21	1,629	97
	s	19	27	1	166	8
Dental periapical	$\bar{x}$	11	344	—	1,110	3
	s	1	58	—	27	1

[a]Different models used to compute marrow dose in each of these studies.
[b]$\bar{x}$ = mean, s = standard error of the mean.
[c]The total energy entering the patient is proportional to the product of the exposure at a point in the beam multiplied by the cross sectional area of the beam at that point.
[d]Please see footnote to Table 10–3 for a discussion of the differences between these two surveys.

Fluoroscopy was initially conducted by directly observing the image produced by the modulated x-ray beam upon a fluorescent screen, called screen fluoroscopy. Dark adaption is required for screen fluoroscopy at reasonable dose rates (~ 3–5 rads per minute). The widespread introduction of the x-ray image intensifier into normal fluoroscopic rooms occurred in the late sixties and early seventies (about a decade after their acceptance for x-ray special procedures).

Image intensifiers provide an image that is several thousand times brighter than the image on the fluoroscopic screen. This bright image permits fluoroscopy under normal ambient lighting at dose rates between 1 and 5 rads per minute. Dark adaption, together with image intensification, does not permit a significant decrease in the dose delivered during fluoroscopy since a certain minimum number of x-ray photons are needed to form a usable image. In general, one can only obtain adequate image quality by using adequate x-ray doses.

The fluoroscopic part of most "fluoroscopic" exams is accompanied by "spot filming." Spot films are radiographs taken to document the patient's anatomy at specific moments during the examination. Most spot films are recorded using conventional radiographic cassettes and radiographic doses. An increasing fraction of such images are obtained by photographing the output of the image intensifier. Due to image quality requirements, such photofluorographs must be made at substantial dose levels.

Fluoroscopic dose levels for typical examinations, as reported by XES-70,[17] are reproduced in Table 4–2. While there is no recent data on fluoroscopic dose rates, image intensification and photofluorographic techniques have probably led to some reduction in doses so that present day examinations are conducted at levels modestly below those shown in Table 4–2.

Angiography

Most angiographic studies can be classified as modified fluoroscopic examinations. Catheters are placed into the patient under fluoroscopic control. Permanent images are recorded at physiologically relevant rates. Film-screen exposures (film changer technique) or photofluorographs are used at imaging rates below 10 images per second. Cinegraphic filming of the image intensifier output is used at higher imaging rates.

Patient doses at the upper end of the diagnostic range are found in angiographic procedures. These doses are due to both the long fluoroscopic times required for catheter placement and to the large number of images needed to demonstrate the anatomy. The relative dose contributions from the fluoroscopic and radiographic components of the study will vary widely from examination to examination. For example, an angioplastic procedure

TABLE 4–2.—REPORTED DOSE FROM FLUOROSCOPIC PROCEDURES*

EXAMINATION	SKIN EXPOSURE RATE (R/min)	MEAN ACTIVE† MARROW DOSE PER EXAMINATION (millirads)	GONADAL DOSE/ PER EXAMINATION† Male (millirads)	Female (millirads)
Barium enema	4.0	875	175	903
Upper GI	4.2	535	1	171
Gallbladder	3.0	168	—‡	78

*XES-70 data.
†Radiographic component.
‡Less than 0.5 millirad/examination

mainly involves fluoroscopy for extensive precision maneuvering of the catheter. A nonselective aortogram, on the other hand, needs little fluoroscopy but requires the production of substantial numbers of full size radiographs.

Cardiac cineangiography is often given as an example of a "high dose" study. It is instructive to dissect the meaning of the concept of "high dose" in this context. A typical study involves the cinematographic filming of contrast media flow in the coronary arteries and in the left ventricle. Fluoroscopy is used to control patient positioning and catheter placement prior to each injection of contrast medium. A study performed by an "average" operator will require 12.7 minutes of fluoroscopy and 110 seconds of cinefluorography.[18] The integral dose in cardiac angiography is minimized by collimating the x-ray beam to the size of the patient's heart. Field sizes below 100 cm^2 are often used (compared to 1,500 cm^2 for a full size radiograph). In addition, the various projections used to demonstrate the coronary arteries irradiate different portions of the patient's skin. These radiographic projections are also designed to minimize the projection of bone images onto the image of the heart. In most projections, both the spine and sternum are excluded from the direct beam. Thus, the effective marrow dose from such a projection is a lower fraction of the skin dose than would be expected for conventional radiography. Although a detailed assessment of the *dose* from cardiac cineangiography is difficult, the overall risk of cardiac angiography may well be comparable with an intravenous pyelogram on the basis of integral dose considerations as well as the volumes of contrast media used.

A newly emerging angiographic modality is *digital fluorography* (DF).[19, 20] Most DF units in clinical use add a digital image processing module to the imaging chain. This module converts the television image into digital form, processes the image to enhance diagnostically useful information and then restores the processed image into analog television format. Digital fluorography requires doses that are higher than fluoroscopy (but lower than angiography) to obtain diagnostic image quality because the process is often used for visualizing low contrast structures.

COMPUTED TOMOGRAPHY (CT)

The production of a CT scan involves measuring the amount of radiation transmitted by each of a large number (about one half million) of small x-ray beams. A computer is subsequently used to reconstruct an image of the tissues through which these beams have passed.

The scanning portion of the CT scanner consists of an x-ray tube with its beam defining collimators and an opposing detector array. In some scanners the detectors form a ring around the patient. In other models, the detectors move in conjunction with the x-ray tube. A thin cross section of tissue (1 to 10 mm) is irradiated as the x-ray tube is moved around the patient. Collimators confine the x-ray beam to this thin section (Fig 4 1).

The patient's skin within this section is uniformly irradiated due to the 360° rotation of the x-ray tube about the patient. Typical skin doses from CT scanning are in the range of 1 to 10 rads. Skin and other tissues a few

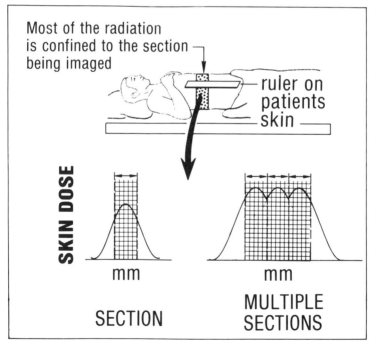

Fig 4–1.—Dose distributions from CT scanning. (See text for explantion.)

millimeters away from the scanned section will not be directly irradiated, but will be exposed to a smaller quantity of radiation scattered from the section. Thus the irradiated tissue is essentially the same tissue which is imaged in the scan. If several adjacent sections are scanned without overlap there will be a small build up of dose from one scan to the next. For present day scanners, the maximum skin dose at the midpoint of a large number of adjacent sections will not be more than 40% greater than the skin dose from a single section.

The integral dose associated with a single CT scan is comparable with the integral dose from a conventional radiograph of the same body part. The integral dose resulting from a series of CT sections is equal to the sum of the integral doses of the individual sections. The collection of CT data is a totally electronic process using sensitive x-ray detectors. The radiologist is relatively free to adjust image quality by adjusting radiation levels. Thus, the quality of the images and the consequential exposure of the patient can be tailored to the purposes of the examination.

RADIONUCLIDE IMAGING

A radionuclide imaging procedure starts by administering a measured amount of the desired radionuclide. The amount of radionuclide administered is described by its activity. The actual amount of the chemical element administered is remarkably small (e.g., 10mCi of ^{99m}Tc has a mass of 2 billionths of a gram). The radioactive tracer mixes with its nonradioactive form or analog and follows the same metabolic pathways as its nonradioactive analog. The radiopharmaceutical (a pharmaceutical containing a radionuclide) is physiologically distributed within the patient. When the atoms of the radionuclide decay they emit both photons and beta particles. Decay energy carried by the beta particles is totally absorbed by the patient and contributes to the patient's dose without contributing to the image. A portion of the decay photons (and photons formed by the annihilation of positive beta particles or positrons) escapes from the patient and can be used for image formation. The nonuniform distribution of radiopharmaceutical in the patient is imaged by observing the nonuniform distribution of photons emitted from the patient.

Desirable properties of radiopharmaceuticals and their underlying radionuclides include: their ability to concentrate in target organs more readily than the rest of the body; zero or minimum decay energy present in the form of nonuseful radiation (i.e., beta particles); reasonable energies for the photons; and rapid clearance after the examination is completed.

As in most imaging cases, one must balance image quality requirements against patient dose. For example, a higher energy gamma photon emitted from a radionuclide will have less chance of being absorbed in the patient but will be more difficult to image properly in an imaging device such as a gamma camera. Furthermore, reducing the administered quantity of radiopharmaceutical will reduce patient dose but may increase examination time and thereby degrade image quality due to increased patient motion.

Table 4–3 indicates the doses received by patients for typical radiopharmaceuticals. The dose to the organs that are imaged will be higher than the whole body doses as a direct consequence of a higher concentration of radionuclide in the target organ.

ULTRASONIC IMAGING

An ultrasonic image is formed by scanning an ultrasonic beam through a section of a patient. As discussed previously, the ultrasonic transducer must be in contact with the patient's skin either directly or via a coupling medium. Reflections from interfaces along the direction of the sound beam are processed by the electronics to form elements of the image. The location of an interface is measured by observing the time required by the sound for its trip from the transducer to the interface. The interface is characterized by the intensity of the echo. The image then is built up by changing the orientation of the sound beam.

Modern ultrasonic apparatus permits the formation of an ultrasonic image either by manually moving the transducer across the patient's skin (compound B scanning) or by automatically moving the sound beam (i.e., linear array scanning, sector scanning). Automatic scanning can be performed at rates compatible with dynamic imaging.

Dosimetry of medical ultrasound requires a totally different set of con-

TABLE 4–3.—ESTIMATED RADIATION ABSORBED DOSE FOR RADIOPHARMACEUTICAL ADMINISTRATION 1978* IN 26 HOSPITALS

| | | AVERAGE ABSORBED RADIATION DOSE PER ADMINISTRATION IN RADS | | | |
RADIONUCLIDE	NUMBER OF ADMINISTRATIONS	WHOLE BODY	GONAD	BONE MARROW	CRITICAL ORGAN
^{131}I	5,569	0.035	0.065	0.078	123.5
^{123}Xe	519	0.035	0.004	0.005	9.2
^{133}Xe	2,807	0.002	0.045	0.001	0.4
^{67}Ga	1,960	1.165	1.165	2.025	4.3
^{201}Tl	694	0.562	1.299	0.772	3.5
^{99}Tc	57,427	0.156	0.154	0.192	4.8
All others	903	1.585	1.700	1.535	4.0
Total	69,879	0.187†	0.199†	0.246†	14.0†

*U.S. Public Health Service unpublished data.
†Weighted average.

cepts from that associated with ionizing radiation. Because ultrasound is a form of nonionizing, nonelectromagnetic radiation, its overall effect will be mechanical damage to tissue. Intercellular effects can be ruled out on the basis that the wavelengths of medical ultrasound (0.1 to 1 mm) are very large relative to cell size.

Mechanical damage to tissue is related to the energy injected into the patient by the ultrasonic beam. Based upon animal experiments, and based upon metabolic energy production in tissue, the American Institute of Ultrasound in Medicine[21] (AIUM) has indicated that an average power level of one hundred milliwatts per square centimeter is safe for long term exposure (~hours). Ultrasonic imaging devices customarily operate at much lower power levels and imaging procedures require shorter exposure times (seconds to minutes). In the authors' opinion, it is highly likely that ultrasonic imaging is safe in an absolute sense.

NUCLEAR MAGNETIC RESONANCE IMAGING

The NMR imaging process involves exposure of the patient to combinations of radio frequency (RF) pulses, stationary and time-varying magnetic fields. While there is as yet little direct information on the hazards of NMR imaging, the hazards of each of these individual electromagnetic fields has been studied. This material was recently reviewed by Budinger.[22] Interim safety standards have been published by the U.S. Public Health Service and by the British National Radiation Protection Board.[23, 24] Formal exposure limits published by these two agencies are shown in Table 4–4.

TABLE 4–4.—SIMPLIFIED INTERIM SAFETY STANDARDS FOR
NUCLEAR MAGNETIC RESONANCE IMAGING (1981–1982)

PATIENT LIMITS	BRH U.S.A. (FEB 82)	NRPB* BRITAIN (NOV 81)	UNITS
Static magnetic field	20,000	25,000	Gauss†
Time varying magnetic field	3,000	20,000 milliseconds or longer	Gauss/Second
Pulsed radio frequency field	0.4/kg whole body	70 whole body	Watts

*National Radiation Protection Board.
†Earth's magnetic field ~ 1 Gauss.

5 / Effects of Ionizing Radiation

OVERVIEW

THERE IS AN ACCEPTED BODY OF INFORMATION describing the effects of high doses of radiation (>100 rads) on man. The predictable effects of very high doses of radiation received by small parts of the body permits precision radiation therapy. While the effects of intermediate doses (10 rads to 100 rads) and low doses (<10 rads) are known in principle, it is increasingly difficult to correlate dose with effect when the dose is lowered. There is, therefore, a great deal of scientific controversy relative to low dose radiation effects. The BEIR-III report was delayed for approximately two years while the somatic effect committee attempted to reach a consensus in this area. The report was finally published without such a consensus being achieved. The BEIR report does present the scope of the disagreement and ranges of radiation effects. Controversy and difficulty arise in large part because radiation effects are relatively rare and are almost totally indistinguishable from natural processes. One therefore attempts to identify radiation effects at dose levels comparable with diagnostic imaging by observing a small, statistically significant increase in disease incidence as a function of radiation dose. This process requires that very large populations be followed for extended periods of time. Webster[25] has calculated that 1,600,000 women would have to be followed for 30 years in order to demonstrate a statistically significant increase in breast cancer following a single high dose (5 rads) mammographic examination. Other major controversial issues include the nature of the dose-effect response, the time course of radiation effects subsequent to an exposure, the nature of the radiation response function (additive or multiplicative), synergistic effects which include a radiation component, etc. A few of these significant points are briefly reviewed in this chapter.

The overall range of effects in man resulting from an acute exposure to radiation is shown in Table 5–1. A complete description of the clinical manifestation of high dose radiation effects is given by Hall.[26] At dose levels exceeding 100,000 millirads (100 rads), radiation effects are said to be nonstochastic (i.e., everyone exposed to such doses will manifest radiation injury and the severity of the individual injury will be proportional to the

TABLE 5–1.—ACUTE RADIATION EFFECTS IN MAN (TOTAL DOSE
RECEIVED IN LESS THAN ONE DAY)

WHOLE BODY DOSE (MILLIRADS)	CRITICAL TISSUE	COMMENT
10,000,000	Central nervous system	Death ~ 1 day
1,000,000	Gastrointestinal mucosa	Death ~ 1 week

Medical treatment becomes effective in reducing the severity of acute effects below 1,000,000 millirads.

600,000	Bone marrow	Possible death ~ 1 month
100,000 "equivalent"	Limited region*	Maximal single radiotherapy treatment
100,000	Bone marrow	Transient white blood cell depression

Medical treatment not required below 20,000 millirads (no acute effects demonstrated).

10,000	Fetus	Increase in congenital abnormalities demonstrated in animals
1,000	Bone marrow	Possible measurable increase in leukemia in adults
1,000	Fetus	Possible statistical increase in tumors resulting from exposure in utero
150	Whole body*	Typical dose from ^{99m}Tc scan
200 "equivalent"	Limited region*	Typical whole body dose "equivalent" from an abdominal radiograph

*For reference purposes, doses resulting from medical procedures are included.

radiation dose received by that individual and that individual's radiosensitivity).

Available information that has been used to quantify the radiation risk resulting from low dose irradiation is derived from epidemiologic studies, animal studies and theoretical radiobiologic studies. Low dose radiation risks are stochastic (the probability of disease incidence is related to the dose, the severity of its expression is unrelated to dose). The best available information is consistent with several models that predict widely different risks at the dose levels used for diagnostic imaging. Because of this divergence of expert opinion, radiation protection guidelines are based upon the most conservative risk model (i.e., the most effect for a given dose).

The evaluation of the radiogenic effect on the incidence of a disease is impeded further by factors such as the usual presence of a latent period after exposure, perhaps a finite period of radiogenic risk and the rising spontaneous incidence of the disease as a function of the patient's age.

Figure 5–1 is a generalized, hypothetical curve showing the radiogenic effect of a single fixed dose irradiation of a population. Such a curve is observed, for example, by following the incidence of leukemia in the Japanese atomic bomb survivors. In general, there will be a period (ranging from a few years to a few decades) after the exposure in which there are no excess cases of the disease relative to an unirradiated control population. This latent period represents the required time for the radiation injury to manifest itself as a clinical disease (i.e., a tumor growing to clinically significant size).

The latent period then is followed by a period in which the irradiated population has a higher incidence of disease than the controls. Demonstrating this increased incidence in a statistically significant manner is often a great challenge. The period of increased incidence in the irradiated population may be followed by a return to the spontaneous incidence implying no radiogenic risk after the period of risk. For leukemia in the Japanese, the latent period was about five years and the period of risk was about 25 years. The period of risk for solid tumors may be the patient's remaining life span.

The nature of the time-risk curve (Fig 5–2) has a profound influence on the prediction of the effect of a single irradiation. The absolute risk model (i.e., the irradiation "will cause" one excess cancer per million people per year) implies extra caution be imposed when irradiating the young. This is

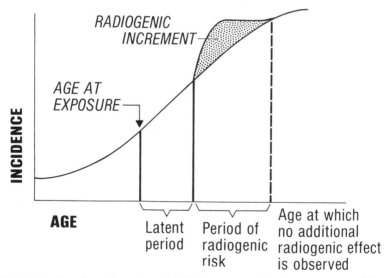

Fig 5–1.—One hypothetical model of the excess risk of carcinogenesis following an exposure to radiation.

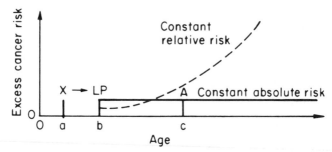

Fig 5–2.—Risk of cancer induction after radiation. The constant absolute *(solid line)* and relative *(broken line)* risk models are plotted against age. a = age at time of irradiation (X); b = age at end of minimal latent period (LP); c = age at a given time after excess cancer risk is expressed. (Used by permission. Fabrikant J.I.[27])

especially true for the model that assumes that the patient is at risk for his remaining life span. The relative risk model (i.e., the irradiation will "double" the patient's chances of cancer) implies extra caution be imposed when irradiating the elderly. This latter conclusion follows from the increase in spontaneous cancer incidence with increasing age.

Assumptions relating to time risk coefficients extrapolated into the future are open to considerable error. One cannot reliably use either model to forecast the risks of irradiation beyond the period of follow up.[27] Perhaps we will have a more detailed time-risk model when the entire population subjected to the atomic bombings have lived out their lives.

The nature of the time effect curve was recently discussed by Gofman.[28] In his opinion, both UNSCEAR and BEIR greatly underestimate the carcinogenic effects of ionizing radiation. Gofman reaches his conclusion by estimating that the period of radiogenic risk from a single exposure may extend until eighty years post exposure. He also assumes that the dose effect curve is gaussian with peak effect expressed forty years post exposure. These assumptions apply a very large cumulative multiplier to risk estimates made with follow up periods shorter than forty or fifty years. In the opinion of the authors of this monograph, Gofman's assumptions may be correct in form and very wrong in numerical estimate of radiation risk.

Gofman proposes an "undoable" experiment; that of exposing a large group of newborns to a single dose of radiation. Lifetime follow up of these individuals' medical histories would then be required to prove the carcinogenic effect of this exposure. In fact, the "undoable" experiment has been done: Newborns have been surgically treated for congenital cardiovascular disease for the past 20 to 30 years. The presurgical angiographic workup of these infants involves tens of rads of essentially whole body irradiation. These patients' spectacular histories of major cardiovascular disease as neonates preclude their loss to follow up. By now there have been enough patient years of follow up so that any evidence that cardiac catheterization (radiation) is a strong carcinogen would have been manifest. The authors are not aware of any studies demonstrating excess cancer in this population. We can therefore conclude that radiation is certainly not as strong a carcinogen as predicted by Gofman.

We have alluded to the problems relating to establishing a dose response curve for low level radiation effects. This difficulty arises from the low radiogenic incidence relative to the spontaneous incidence of most diseases at low dose levels. A generalized experimental dose response curve is shown on the right hand side of Figure 5–3. The uncertainty in the risk due to any given dose rises as the dose decreases. The shaded area represents the region associated with diagnostic imaging (the low level region). The shaded region also represents the area of greatest scientific uncertainty relative to the form of the dose response function.

The mechanism by which radiation induces a carcinogenic change in tissue is related to ionization damage of chromosomes and DNA. Different theoretical models may be derived based upon the linear energy transfer (LET) of the radiation and upon its dose rate. The reader is referred to any of the standard radiobiology texts such as Hall[26] or Pizzarello[29] for further information.

The two principal theoretical models for the low level dose response function for x-rays are the pure linear and the linear quadratic. A third general function discussed by the BEIR report is the pure quadratic. This

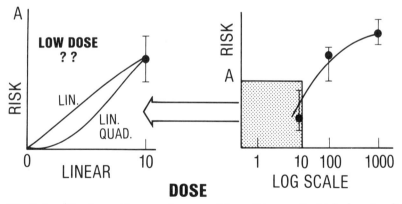

Fig 5–3.—The dose-risk curve is reasonably well-known for high dose irradiations. There is considerable experimental and epidemiologic uncertainty for dose levels corresponding to diagnostic radiology. Even the shape of the dose-risk curve is unknown at low doses. Two dose-response models discussed by the BEIR Report are shown. LIN. = linear; LIN. QUAD. = linear quadratic.

latter form is likely to be of little relevance to diagnostic x-ray imaging. The general form of the first two functions is shown on the left-hand side of Figure 5–3. Both models assume the absence of a threshold dose. Thus any radiation exposure is assumed to have an associated risk (even background radiation!). The linear model assumes that if a radiation interaction produces damage, the damage will result in injury. The linear quadratic model assumes that some fraction of radiation interactions will produce direct injury and that another fraction will produce subinjurious damage. In this model, the higher the dose the more likely that several subinjurious interactions will combine to produce an injury and hence the superlinear increase in risk with increasing dose. (Superlinear describes a function which increases more rapidly than a straight line as its argument is increased.)

Because it is so conservative, the zero threshold linear dose response function has been the basis of radiologic risk assessment for the past decades. The conservative nature of this model is customarily strengthened by assuming that there is no biologic repair of radiation injuries. As such, it represents a worst case model for predicting the radiologic risks of diagnostic imaging.

The linear quadratic model of the dose response function is taken to be a probable model for somatic risk by the majority of the Committee on the Biological Effects of Ionizing Radiation (BEIR-III).[30] It represents a generalized form of the dose response function and appears to fit some experimental and epidemiologic data better than the pure linear model. To the extent to which the linear quadratic model better represents the available data than does the pure linear model, the actual risk from diagnostic imaging will be lower.

Although to remain conservative we will use the linear, zero threshold, zero repair model in the remainder of this report, it is instructive to review one of many calculations performed by the BEIR-III committee. Table 5–2 reproduces an overall risk calculation which demonstrates the influence of dose response models and time response models on the estimate of the risk resulting from a single substantial exposure. Note that, depending upon the model selected, the numeric value of the risk can vary over a range in excess of fifty to one.

We can simplify by extrapolating to 100 millirads per year resulting from the use of diagnostic imaging and an absolute risk model. One then arrives at the conclusion that the net risk is an increase in the cancer mortality ranging from 0.5% [linear model] to 0.1% [linear quadratic model]. Thus, one can estimate, using BEIR-III figures, that cancer mortality in the U.S. resulting from diagnostic radiology is below 1,000 individuals per year (compared to 50,000 deaths per year due to automobile accidents). Hall[31]

TABLE 5–2.—Excess Mortality per Million
Persons from All Forms
of Cancer* After a Single Whole Body
10 Rad X-Ray Dose

DOSE RESPONSE MODEL	EXCESS DEATHS AS % OF NORMAL†	
	PROJECTION MODEL	
	ABSOLUTE RISK	RELATIVE RISK
Linear	1.0	3.1
Linear-Quadratic	0.47	1.4
Quadratic	0.058	0.17

*Adapted from Table V-23 BEIR-III. Used by permission.
†Normal expectation 163,800 cancer deaths per million population.

estimates that there are between 1,000 and 4,000 radiogenic cancer deaths per year in the United States for a per capita dose rate of 0.1 rem per year.

The BEIR report gives the results of calculations that are age and sex selective, model selective, dose rate selective and disease selective. The reader is referred to the original document for further details. One should note that while order of magnitude calculations of low level radiation risks are possible, it is unlikely that sufficient human data will ever be available so that one could quantify the risk more accurately than ± 50%.

SOMATIC EFFECTS AT DIAGNOSTIC DOSE LEVELS

Radiation-Induced Aging

One of the postulated nonstochastic effects of radiation is a nonspecific life shortening called radiation-induced aging. This question originally arose as a consequence of the untimely deaths of many early radiation workers (Fig 5–4). These workers received doses at rates estimated to exceed 1,000 rads per year. In addition, Mettler's[32] report on the work of the United Nations Scientific Committee on the Effects of Atomic Radiation (UNSCEAR)[33] includes the statement that in the mouse there is a linear relationship between acute irradiation and life shortening. The reduction in life span in the mouse is 5% per 100 rads whole body, down to the lowest doses. However, this long-term life shortening by radiation may be reasonably accounted for by an increased incidence of neoplastic conditions taking some of the animals to a premature death (statements paraphrased for brevity).

There have been extensive investigations into the mortality of American radiologists indicating some excess mortality among the radiologists.[34, 35]

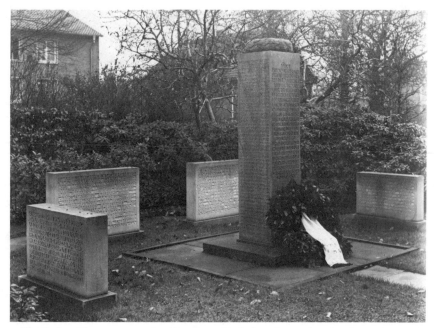

Fig 5–4.—Monument to the Martyrs of Radiology located in St. Georg Hospital, Hamburg, West Germany. (Courtesy of CHF Müller, Hamburg.)

This effect appears to be due to an increased incidence of neoplasm in the older radiologists (these individuals were in practice prior to World War II and may be presumed to have received much higher doses than present practice permits). A study of Army x-ray technologists by Jablon and Miller[36] indicated no excess mortality in this group relative to other military medical technologists. The follow up of the Japanese atomic bomb survivors has demonstrated no increase in non-neoplastic mortality.[37] The hypothesis of a nonstochastic radiation-induced aging does not hold up against the available evidence. One can therefore conclude that actuarial life shortening in an irradiated population is due to the appearance of neoplasm (a stochastic effect) in a fraction of that population.

Fertility Effects

The impairment of fertility by radiation is a nonstochastic cell killing effect. Permanent sterilizing doses are about 500 rads for an acute exposure and about 1,500 rads fractionated over a few days.

In the male, fertility can be impaired by acute testicular doses of 100 rads. This damage is repaired by repopulation of the seminiferous epithelium by surviving spermatogonial cells.

In the female, an acute ovarian dose in the range 300 to 400 rads is required to impair fertility. This higher dose is required by the relative radioresistance of resting human oocytes. Fertility is restored by the maturing of a surviving oocyte. The dose required for permanent sterilization decreases with age due to physiologic atresia of the oocytes.

Cataracts

The radiogenic induction of cataracts is a nonstochastic process. Merriam and Focht[38] performed an extensive investigation into the induction of radiogenic cataracts as a side effect of radiotherapy. They found that the threshold dose for cataract formation is 200 rads for x-rays given acutely. The minimum lens doses associated with radiogenic cataracts increased with dose fractionation. A threshold of 550 rads was found for doses fractionated over one month.

An acute threshold of 200 rads is consistent with the Nagasaki experience. Lower thresholds are found for heavy particle irradiation in man and for x-ray exposure in rodents.

Cancer Induction

The knowledge of the carcinogenic properties of ionizing radiation dates back to the early years of the twentieth century. Most of the "Martyrs to Radiology" died of radiogenic malignancy. This was certainly caused by the massive doses received by these individuals.

The carcinogenic potentials associated with low levels of radiation have been investigated in the years following World War II. Human studies include the radiation effects on the Japanese atomic bomb survivors as well as groups of irradiated patients. Innumerable animal experiments dealing with the genetic and carcinogenic effects of low levels of radiation have been conducted over the past four decades. The scale of the animal experiments has ranged from a few specimens to the "megamouse" experiments conducted at Oak Ridge in the early 1960s. (A megamouse experiment is a study using one million mice as experimental subjects.) It is not surprising therefore to find that most hard data on low level radiation effects is based upon small animal experience. Human data is mainly epidemiologic and in most cases based upon retrospective epidemiology. The uncertainties of using either the sparse direct human data or transferring animal experience to man makes the study of radiation carcinogenesis difficult.

The BEIR Committee has categorized the carcinogenic effects of ionizing radiation on different tissues.[39] Their review is reproduced in Table 5–3. The data demonstrate both age and site selective components of radiogenic risk. While the general trend of the data is clear, assessment of numeric risks is highly dependent upon the dose-risk model used for the calculations. The epidemiologic evidence supporting this data comes from the

TABLE 5-3.—SENSITIVITY OF VARIOUS TISSUES TO CARCINOGENIC INDUCTION BY RADIATION*

SITE OR TYPE OF CANCER	SPONTANEOUS INCIDENCE OF CANCER	RELATIVE SENSITIVITY TO RADIATION INDUCTION OF CANCER	REMARKS
Major radiation-induced cancers			
Female breast	Very high	High	Puberty increases sensitivity
Thyroid	Low	Very high, especially females	Low mortality rate
Lung (bronchus)	Very high	Moderate	Quantitative effect of smoking uncertain
Leukemia	Moderate	Very high	Especially myeloid leukemia
Alimentary tract	High	Moderate to low	Occurs especially in colon
Minor radiation-induced cancers			
Pharynx	Low	Moderate	—
Liver and biliary tract	Low	Moderate	—
Pancreas	Moderate	Moderate	
Lymphomas	Moderate	Moderate	Lymphosarcoma and multiple myeloma, but not Hodgkin's disease
Kidney and bladder	Moderate	Low	—
Brain and nervous system	Low	Low	—
Salivary glands	Very low	Low	
Bone	Very low	Low	
Skin	High	Low	Low mortality. High dose necessary?
Sites or tissues in which magnitude of radiation-induced cancer is uncertain			
Larynx	Moderate	Low	
Nasal sinuses	Very low	Low	
Parathyroid	Very low	Low	
Ovary	Moderate	Low	
Connective tissues	Very low	Low	
Sites or tissues in which radiation-induced cancer has not been observed			
Prostate	Very high	Absent?	
Uterus and cervix	Very high	Absent?	
Testis	Low	Absent?	
Mesentery and mesothelium	Very low	Absent?	
Chronic lymphatic leukemia	Low	Absent?	

*From BEIR-III report. Used by permission.

study of small groups (summarized in Table 5–4). It should also be noted that many of these groups were irradiated for the purpose of treating another illness.

There are long latent periods associated with most radiogenic cancers. These latent periods were reviewed by the UNSCEAR[40] Committee and are summarized in Table 5–5.

FETAL EFFECTS

The irradiated fetus faces two broad classes of risk: a nonstochastic risk of developmental defects and a stochastic risk of radiogenic neoplasm. We will briefly review these two topics in this section.

Nonstochastic effects in the irradiated fetus occur at dose levels (~5 rads) which are below that required to produce an effect in the adult (~100 rads). The additional sensitivity of fetal cells to radiation is related to their rapid differentiation and division. Thus, specific damage will be induced when a fetus is irradiated at a specific point in its developmental cycle. Rugh[41] has reported extensive experimental evidence documenting the induction of specific abnormalities in the mouse. Figure 5–5 summarizes these events.

Irradiation damage to the fetus was recently reviewed by L. Russell.[42] As reviewed by Russell, and as indicated in Figure 5–5, radiation effects may be divided into preimplantation, major organogenesis and fetal growth

TABLE 5–4.—REASON FOR IRRADIATION OF
SOME OF THE POPULATIONS USED BY BEIR
FOR RADIATION RISK ESTIMATES

Female breast 269–288*	Multiple fluoroscopy (several hundred low dose fractions). Fluoroscopic control of therapeutic pneumothorax for tuberculosis.
	Post partum mastitis (few high dose fractions)—radiation therapy.
	Atomic bomb survivors (single exposure).
Thyroid 288–307*	Tinea capitis—radiation therapy
	Thymic enlargement—radiation therapy
	Hydrogen bomb fallout
	Atomic bomb survivors
Lung 308–331*	Ankylosing spondylitis—radiation therapy
	Atomic bomb survivors
	Uranium miners
Leukemia 331–357*	Atomic bomb survivors
	Ankylosing spondylitis—radiation therapy
	U.S. radiologists—prior to 1930
Alimentary tract 357–372*	Atomic bomb survivors
	Ankylosing spondylitis—radiation therapy

*Pages in BEIR-III report.

TABLE 5–5.—Examples of Long Mean Latencies
Recorded Following Therapeutic Radiation*

NUMBER OF SUBJECTS	SITE OF CANCER	MEAN LATENCY (YEARS)
20	Thyroid	20.3
10	Bladder	20.7
10	Breast	22.6
9	Various, on head and neck	22.8
37	Pharynx and larynx	23.4
113	Various, on head and neck	24.1
38	Skin	24.5
10	Pharynx	25.0
130	Pharynx and larynx	27.3
40	Skin (basal cell)	41.5

*From UNSCEAR. Used by permission.

phases. Radiation injury during the preimplantation stage will generally cause embryonic death. Radiation injury during the major organogenesis phase can give rise to most of the congenital abnormalities as shown in Figure 5–5. The exact abnormality is dependent on the tissues at risk during the time of irradiation. Radiation injury during the fetal growth phase may cause cell depletion with a consequent reduction in organ size.

Because of the relatively long fraction of the human gestation cycle occupied by neural development, there is specific concern relative to both gross and subtle radiogenic neurologic disease. Russell's review reports specific effects in this area.

The general dose reponse curve for fetal irradiation is thought to be sigmoidal with a threshold dose, ranging from below 5 rads to above 100 rads, depending upon fetal age and the specific injury. Radiogenic malformations are generally indistinguishable from spontaneous malformations. It may therefore be impossible to determine the true radiogenic incidence of malformations at fetal dose ranges comparable with ordinary diagnostic imaging ($<$ 10 rads).

The second broad range of fetal risk is the susceptibility of the fetus, and perhaps the unfertilized mature oocyte, to radiogenic leukemia.[43–46] Retrospective studies indicate that in utero irradiation at dose levels of one rad may double the risk of leukemia during the first decade of life. These studies have been extensively reviewed in the BEIR-III report[47] without a firm conclusion being drawn but including a summary ending with: "The period of increased risk appears to begin at birth and last for 12 years for hematopoietic tumors and about 10 years for solid tumors, with parallel risk coefficients of 25 excess fatal leukemias per million children per year per

X-IRRADIATION-INDUCED CONGENITAL ANOMALIES

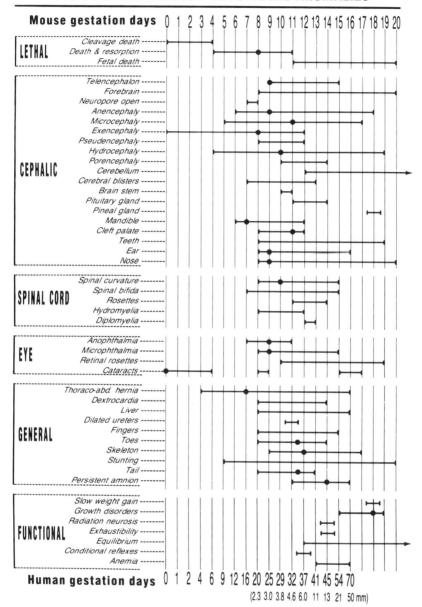

Fig 5–5.—Summarized data on the congenital effects of ionizing radiations on the embryo or fetus of nonhuman mammals. This figure illustrates the embryonic period when a particular organ is likely to be affected. The time of maximum susceptibility is indicated by a large dot and the bars indicate the range of time over which the anomaly has been observed. The scale at the bottom gives comparable ages for human embryos. (From Rugh R.[41] Used by permission.)

rad and 28 excess fatal cancers of other types." Webster,[25] in his review of the BEIR report, regards the greater sensitivity of the fetus to be unsubstantiated.

GENETIC EFFECTS

The mutagenic capacity of ionizing radiation has been known for the past half century. The genetic effects of radiation were reported by H. J. Muller[48] in 1927. This work was brought to the public's attention in the years immediately following World War II.[49] The concept of stochastic risk was first developed as an explanation of radiation mutagenesis. Sources of genetically significant radiation doses are shown in Table 5–6.

The interaction of a single photon of ionizing radiation with tissue releases enough energy within a small volume so as to disrupt molecular bonds. Such interactions occurring in a chromosome can destroy a single gene or cause a chromosomal breakage or dislocation. A model of radiation mutagenesis which is a linear function of dose, has zero threshold dose and assumes no repair of radiation damage, is therefore appropriate.

The expression of a radiogenic mutation requires its transmission to the

TABLE 5–6.—SOURCES OF GENETICALLY SIGNIFICANT
RADIATION DOSES*

SOURCE	DOSE EQUIVALENT RATE (millirems/yr)
Natural radiation	
Cosmic radiation	28
Radionuclides in the body	28
External gamma radiation from terrestrial sources	26
Subtotal	82
Man-made radiation	
Medical and dental x-rays	
Patients	20
Occupational	<0.4
Radiopharmaceuticals	
Patients	2–4
Occupational	<0.15
Commercial nuclear power	
Environment	<1
Occupational	<0.15
National laboratories and contractors—occupational	<0.2
Industrial application—occupational	<0.01
Military applications—occupational	<0.04
Weapons—testing fallout	4–5
Consumer products	4–5
Air travel	<0.5
Subtotal	30–40 (approx.)

*BEIR-III Report. Used by permission.

offspring of the irradiated parent. A fraction of the effects will appear in the first generation after irradiation. The remaining portion will be expressed in subsequent generations. As radiogenic mutations do not differ from spontaneous mutations, one is faced with the problem of detecting a small increment on a substantial background. The Drosophila and Oak Ridge megamouse experiments were helpful in this respect but only give indirect evidence as to the human situation. The atomic bomb survivors represent the largest irradiated group in which one can look for genetic effects. This group has been recently reappraised by Shull et al.[50]

The mutagenic effects of radiation may be quantified in terms of a "doubling dose." This is the quantity of radiation that will induce a mutation rate twice the spontaneous mutation rate. By mathematical techniques, it can be shown that if all spontaneous mutations are due to background radiation, then the doubling dose is 3 rads. The BEIR Committee[51] has estimated the doubling dose in man to be in the range of 50 to 250 rads. The UNSCEAR report suggests "that the doubling dose in man (both sexes) is unlikely to be lower than 100 rads." The evaluation of the Japanese experience by Shull et al. yields an average doubling dose of 156 rem under conditions of the bombing.

The megamouse experiments have demonstrated sexual differences, dose rate effects and biorepair of radiation-induced mutagenesis. The germinal cells at risk are the spermatogonia and the oocytes. Both experimental results and theoretic radiobiology demonstrate a substantially lesser sensitivity of the oocytes relative to the spermatogonia. (The oocytes are dormant, but the spermatogonia undergo cell division; hence the greater radiosensitivity of the latter).

The doubling dose in the female is estimated to be at least 40% higher than in the male and may exceed twice the male value. Most of the human genetic risk of exposure to radiation therefore is borne by the exposure of prospective fathers. Mother Nature thus seems to be protecting her own since ovarian shielding during abdominal x-ray examinations is not usually feasible.

Animal experiments have demonstrated a decrease in the mutagenic ability of radiation as the dose rate is lowered toward 800 millirads per minute. Diagnostic x-ray exposures, which include the gonads in the direct beam, are delivered at gonadal dose rates which can exceed 10,000 millirads per minute. Examinations of other body parts will deliver low gonadal doses at low dose rates. Thus, the relative mutagenic effect of diagnostic x-rays may vary over a wide range as a complex function of examination technique.

The repair of genetic damage can be simply pictured as the bioelimination of damaged gametes prior to conception. Animal experiments have demonstrated a reduction in mutation rate by providing a time interval of a few months between irradiation and conception.

One can estimate the number of genetic diseases induced into the population from the practice of diagnostic radiology. The genetically significant dose resulting from diagnostic imaging procedures is 24 millirads per year or 720 millirads per generation.[52] For 1,000 millirads per generation and a doubling dose of 100 rads, UNSCEAR calculates that in the first generation there will be a 0.06 percent increase in genetic disease.[33] The effect of irradiating the population at that dose level for many generations will be a radiogenic increment of 0.17% above the spontaneous rate of genetic disease.

6 / Effects of Nonionizing Radiation

ULTRASOUND

THE POSSIBILITY OF TISSUE DAMAGE as a consequence of its irradiation by diagnostic ultrasound beams is still open. Several publications in the literature report adverse effects resulting from ultrasonic irradiation. Unfortunately, the variety of findings reported in these publications have not been reproducible or consistent from investigator to investigator. Therefore, we will bypass the anecdotal evidence and discuss the bioeffects of ultrasonic imaging in a categorical manner.

There are three major mechanisms by which ultrasound can damage tissue. These are ultrasonic heating, cavitation and mechanical effects. Heating will depend upon the average flow of energy into the patient. Cavitation is the formation of microbubbles in the ultrasonically irradiated medium. It is a function of the instantaneous peak intensity of the sound beam and its frequency. Mechanical effects, if they occur, are probably caused by resonances between ultrasonic waves and organized tissue elements of similar size (0.1 to 1 mm).

There has been a great deal of experimental investigation into the bioeffects of ultrasound.[53–55] The American Institute of Ultrasound in Medicine[21] formulated the following statement on the biological risks of ultrasound.

> "Statement on Mammalian In Vivo Ultrasonic Biological Effects"
> August 1976

> "In the low megahertz frequency range there have been (as of this date) no demonstrated significant biological effects in mammalian tissues exposed to intensities* below 100 mW/cm². Furthermore, for ultrasonic exposure times** less than 500 seconds and greater than one second, such effects have not been demonstrated even at higher intensities, when the product of intensity* and exposure time** is less than 50 joules/cm².

Kremkau[56] has compared this statement with the known outputs of diagnostic ultrasonic instruments. Figure 6–1 demonstrates this comparison.

---

*Spatial peak, temporal average as measured in a free field in water.
**Total time; this includes off-time as well as on-time for a repeated-pulse regimen."

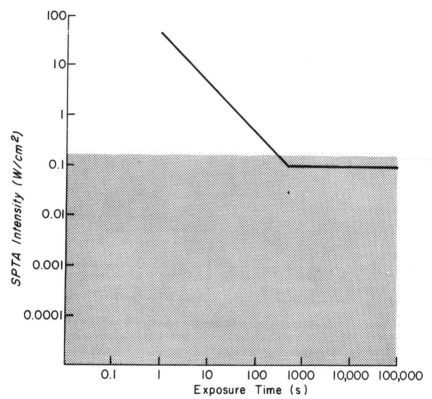

Fig 6–1.—Comparison of instrument output data with AIUM bioeffects statement level. The dark line represents the AIUM Guideline (levels below this line are presumed to be safe). The shaded area shows the range in which diagnostic instruments fall. Spatial peak temporal average (SPTA) intensity is used, assuming that temporal average is relevant. Time is total time of exposure to ultrasound (includes time between pulses in the case of pulsed ultrasound). (From Kremkau F.W.[56] Used by permission.)

To the extent at which one can compare risks by means of average power, it appears that diagnostic ultrasound is safe. The question of cavitation effects relating to peak power (a SPTA value of 100 milliwatts per square centimeter corresponds to a peak power of 10 watts per square centimeter) or resonance effects is still open. Ultrasonographers should therefore operate their equipment at minimal power levels.

NUCLEAR MAGNETIC RESONANCE

The fields used in NMR imaging are the static magnetic field, the time varying magnetic field, and the pulsed radiofrequency field. The effects of radiofrequency fields on humans are the best understood of these fields used in NMR imaging. The radio frequencies used for NMR imaging have wavelengths in the range from 1 to 100 meters. These wavelengths are not microwaves. Thus the RF exposure hazard is related to direct tissue heating (similar to short wave diathermy). The interim standards limit the heating effect of the RF fields to a value approximating the patient's basal metabolic rates. This is well below the patient's ability to heat his own tissues by exercise.

Induced voltages and currents are the primary concerns relative to both the static and time varying magnetic fields. While a catalog of such eventualities was discussed by Buddinger,[22] his review of the literature yielded no consistent evidence of hazard at the magnetic field strengths used for NMR imaging. More research is needed in this area.

Anecdotally, the main reported hazard of NMR images has been to the experimenters' magnetic stripe credit cards, watches and tools. There are real unanswered questions relating to the magnetic environment of NMR imaging machines. The influence of the environment (i.e., moving automobiles or equipment carts) on image quality as well as the fringing magnetic fields of the imager on passers by (i.e., on pacemakers) needs careful attention.

7 / Selection of Patients and Examinations

AS NEWER IMAGING MODALITIES ARE INTRODUCED and information regarding their efficacy is discovered, communication between the radiologist and the clinician is essential. The clinician and radiologist must not only consider the value of the procedure in determining a diagnosis but how this procedure may be performed with the least expenditure of risk and dollars. It must be pointed out that the risk of radiation in many instances is much less than other risks of the procedure. As stated earlier, the risk of death from contrast injection is significant: 1 death per 5,000 in intravenous cholangiography[1]; 1 death in 96,000 intravenous pyelograms.[2] There are recognized complications of the more invasive procedures. It is imperative that the radiologist performs his or her role as a consultant, then, in helping to select the diagnostic procedures considering all the factors.

As stated in the introduction, it is impossible in this book to direct the clinician in every clinical situation in selecting the examination for the patient or the patient for the examination. On the other hand, there is clear indication in certain clinical settings that specific examinations or combinations of examinations are more likely to yield a significant answer than others, always bearing in mind the desire of minimizing radiation dose in achieving this goal. BRH has published some general guides on the selection of patients.[57–59] In addition, there are certain examinations that are clearly overutilized and examinations that are performed which yield no significant information. Emphasis will be placed on these clinical situations.

Most of the high dose examinations are abdominal and the majority of the radiosensitive organs (i.e., bone marrow, ovaries, uterus [fetus], testicles) are maximally exposed by abdominal radiography. We will therefore emphasize some symptom/sign complexes or clinical suspicions of a specific disease in the abdomen.

With the advent of newer imaging modalities, in many cases a high dose conventional examination or even several high dose examinations can be eliminated with the use of one of these newer procedures. For example, the dose from a single CT examination would be less than the several conventional procedures it replaces.

THE NEW YORK HOSPITAL ALGORITHMS

Some algorithms have evolved at The New York Hospital[60] based on our experience with the newer imaging modalities as well as with conventional procedures. It must be stressed that different approaches may be used at different institutions based on their experience and expertise. For didactic purposes only, Figure 7–1 illustrates the most common abdominal radiologic procedures and the grossly comparative radiation "skin dose" a patient might receive from each procedure. The actual dose and dose distribution associated with any given examination will vary widely from facility to facility and from patient to patient. Based on the discussion of dose distribution in Chapter 3 (Figs 3–1 and 3–2), the provision of the simplified "skin dose" chart shown in Figure 7–1 must be recognized as a teaching

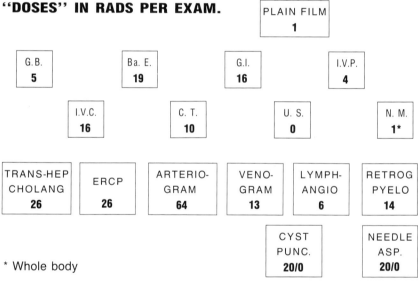

"DOSES" IN RADS PER EXAM.

Fig 7–1.—Our estimate of approximate "skin doses" for abdominal imaging procedures. These values are used only for gross comparisons in the following examples. (See text for a review of dosimetric concepts.) Actual dose and dose distributions for any given examination will vary widely from facility to facility and from patient to patient. G.B. = cholecystogram; Ba.E. = barium enema; G.I. = gastrointestinal series; I.V.P. = intravenous pyelogram; I.V.C. = study of the inferior vena cava; C.T. = computerized tomography; U.S. = ultrasound; N.M. = nuclear medicine radionuclide scan; TRANS-HEP CHOLANG = transhepatic cholangiogram; ERCP = endoscopic retrograde cholangiopancreatography; LYMPHANGIO = lymphangiogram; RETROG PYELO = retrograde pyelogram; CYST PUNC. = cyst puncture (20 rads if fluoroscopy is used, no radiation if ultrasound is used); NEEDLE ASP = needle aspiration.

aid only. The same caveat applies to Tables 7–1 to 7–7. If necessary the entrance skin exposure can be estimated by using the data given in Appendix B. If an accurate dose estimate is required then the examination circumstances will have to be evaluated by an expert in radiation dosimetry.

Retroperitoneal Adenopathy

In the selection of an examination, consideration must be given to the radiation dose as well as to the invasiveness of the procedure, the cost of the examination and how much additional information beyond lymph node evaluation will be obtained (i.e., tumor involvement of the liver, spleen, etc.).

Evaluation of retroperitoneal lymph node lesions happily has advanced from the use of insensitive modalities and modalities with a relatively high dose of radiation such as barium studies, intravenous pyelograms and examinations of the inferior vena cava to more accurate methods such as lymphangiography, CT scanning and ultrasound. Using one or even several of these modalities yields considerably more information than the evaluations entailing previously mentioned procedures, and at a significant "savings" in rads (Table 6–1).

Lymphangiography has the advantage of visualizing the lymph node architecture, and then may diagnose disease in a nonenlarged node or may declare "normal" an enlarged hyperplastic node. On the other hand, this procedure only evaluates para-aortic, vena cava, common and external iliac nodes. CT screening can visualize any enlarged intra-abdominal lymph nodes. In addition, unlike lymphangiography, the visualization of tumor involvement of other viscera is possible. CT however cannot detect tumor involvement in a nonenlarged lymph node. We recommend CT as the initial procedure for evaluating retroperitoneal lymph node involvement, particularly in diseases expected to enlarge nodes if involved and reserve lymphangiography for patients with negative CT. Occasionally ultrasound is valuable in very thin patients but does not visualize all the retroperitoneum because of overlying gas. Our approach is illustrated in Figure 7–2. Table 7–1 shows the radiation exposure using CT with or without lymphangiography compared to the classic work-up without access to CT.

TABLE 7–1.—RETROPERITONEAL ADENOPATHY*

	DOSE
a) CT	10 Rads
b) CT, Lymph.	14 Rads
c) GI, BaE, IVP	39 Rads
d) CT, Lymph, GI, BaE, IVP	53 Rads

*See Fig 7–1 for legend and caveat.

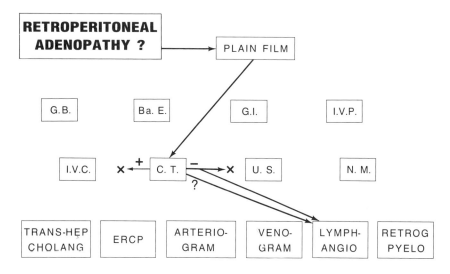

X = STOP

Fig 7–2.—Diagnostic approach to retroperitoneal adenopathy. Previously used procedures such as excretory urography (intravenous pyelography, I.V.P.) and barium studies (Ba.E., G.I.) are now bypassed in favor of a CT examination. The plain film is helpful, though not essential, in the interpretation of any sectional imaging or tomographic procedure. Lymphangiography is recommended routinely after equivocal, or negative CT studies. Ultrasound (U.S.) has been useful as a supplement to CT in very thin patients.

Abdominal Aortic Aneurysm

It is not an uncommon problem for a clinician to palpate a pulsatile abdominal mass and not be able to differentiate a tortuous aorta, an aortic aneurysm or a mass adjacent to a pulsatile aorta. Ultrasound now offers a simple, inexpensive solution without ionizing radiation. This replaces other time honored procedures such as abdominal films (usually AP, lateral and obliques), IVPs and even barium studies. Figure 7–3 illustrates our approach at The New York Hospital. CT is reserved for cases where, because of overlying gas, the distal aorta and bifurcation cannot be visualized. An aortogram may or may not be done prior to surgery, depending on the desires of the surgeon.

Renal Mass

A not uncommon clinical problem is the detection of a mass in the kidney either because of symptoms such as hematuria or on a radiographic finding on a urogram done for other reasons or even on an incidental finding on another type of radiographic examination. The great majority of cys-

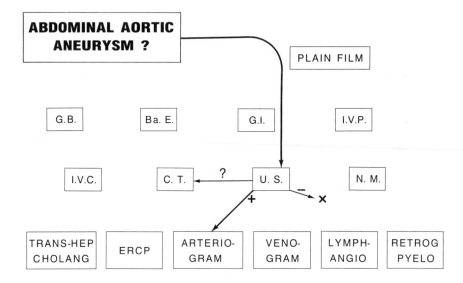

X=STOP

Fig 7–3.—Diagnostic approach for suspected abdominal aortic aneurysm. Ultrasound is initial procedure of choice. No further imaging studies are indicated after an unequivocally negative sonogram. CT is performed if portions of aorta are obscured by gas or fat. Aortography may be performed prior to surgery.

tic renal masses are benign, while most solid masses are malignant. Prior to sonography, angiography was required for the differentiation of a solid, vascular mass from a cystic one as nephrotomography is not always definitive. Sonography is more definitive than angiography in differentiating cystic from avascular masses. In certain cases, angiography is required and CT may supplement the ultrasound diagnosis. Sonography, however, is the initial radiographic procedure and often the only imaging procedure done. If the ultrasound examination unequivocally diagnoses a cyst in an asymptomatic individual over 50 years of age, no other procedure is done. If symptomatic, a cyst puncture may be required. See Figure 7–4 for our diagnostic approach and Table 7–2 for the radiation dose for this approach or variations of that approach, using other modalities.

Nonfunctioning Kidney

The initial step in the evaluation of a unilateral or bilateral nonfunctioning kidney is to determine if the cause is due to obstruction or renal parenchymal disease. In the past retrograde pyelography was normally done, but ultrasound can now make this differential diagnosis with a high degree of certainty. A completely normal sonogram essentially excludes obstruction as a cause of nonfunction, precluding the need of a retrograde pyelogram. A radionuclide scan can be performed if renovascular disease or transplant rejection is suspected. Angiography can be carried out to diagnose arterial or venous disease.

A retrograde pyelogram can be done to localize the precise site of obstruction diagnosed by ultrasound. In equivocal cases on ultrasound, CT scanning may be of great benefit. We then use ultrasound as the primary tool in evaluating nonfunctioning kidneys (Fig 7–5).

Adrenal Mass

Due to its small size and being adjacent to much larger organs, the radiologic evaluation of the adrenal gland was extremely difficult prior to the introduction of ultrasound and CT scanning. Adding to this difficulty is that pathologic enlargement of the adrenal is often quite small. CT has made it possible to easily evaluate the adrenal glands and is used by us as the first

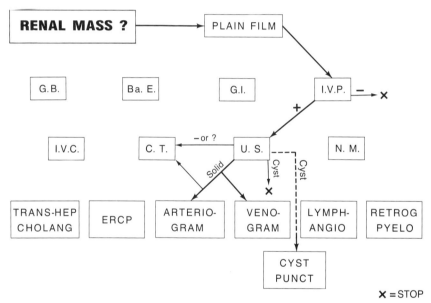

Fig 7–4.—Diagnostic approach to renal masses. Ultrasound is performed first for masses suspected on excretory urography (I.V.P.). If mass is unequivocally cystic on sonography, confirmatory cyst puncture is performed only for younger patients (under 50 years) or if there are signs or symptoms suggesting neoplasm or abscess. Otherwise, cystic mass is followed by ultrasound at progressively increasing intervals. CT is valuable for masses which are equivocal or not shown on sonography and in certain other clinical situations, for example, angiomyolipoma vs. clear cell hypernephroma, acute abscess or hematoma, extent of disease. Angiography is routinely performed preoperatively.

TABLE 7–2.—RENAL MASS*

	DOSE
a) IVP, US	4 Rads
b) IVP, US, Cyst Punct.	2 4/4 Rads†
c) IVP, US, CT	14 Rads
d) IVP, US, Art., Veno	81 Rads
e) IVP, US, CT, Art., Veno	91 Rads

*See Fig 7–1 for legend and caveat.
†The dose is 24 rads if the cyst puncture is performed under fluoroscopic control; it will be 4 rads if it is performed under ultrasonic control.

radiologic procedure. It has largely replaced angiography. Ultrasound is used as a supplement to further evaluate the internal structure of masses demonstrated on CT or in very thin patients. Small adenomas, usually associated with aldosteronism, may be missed on CT and may require venography or venous sampling. Our approach is summarized in Figure 7–6.

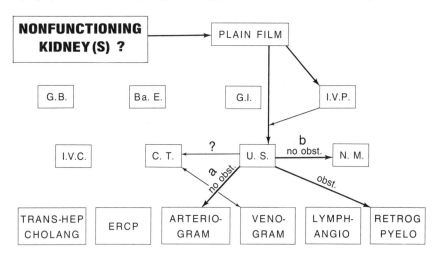

a = Suspected artery or venous obstruction.

b = Suspected renovascular abnormality.

Fig 7–5.—Diagnostic approach to nonfunctioning kidney(s). Nonfunction may be discovered on excretory urography (I.V.P.) or patient may be azotemic. In the latter case, plain film is useful, especially to look for calcifications. Totally normal ultrasound with no distortion of renal landmarks excludes obstruction as cause of nonfunction. Radionuclide scan (N.M. = nuclear medicine) or angiography may then be performed if indicated clinically. CT is useful when kidney and adjacent structures are not delineated on sonography. Retrograde pyelography (RETROG PYELO) generally performed when pyelocaliectasis is shown on ultrasound.

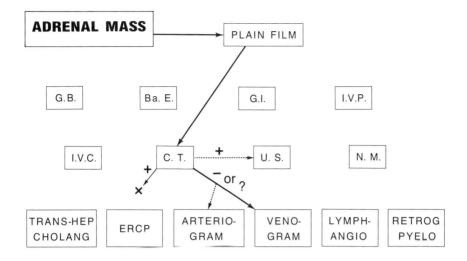

Fig 7–6.—Diagnostic approach to adrenal masses. CT is initial procedure of choice. No further imaging studies necessary after unequivocally positive CT. Angiography, especially venography with hormonal assays, is performed routinely after negative or equivocal CT. Ultrasound is useful as supplement to CT for studying the internal structure of an adrenal mass or in very thin patients with abnormal CT. Iodocholesterol nuclear medicine scans (N.M.) may provide valuable functional information in some cases.

Pancreas

The selection of an imaging procedure for the pancreas is extremely complex since there are multiple types of pancreatic diseases, both neoplastic and inflammatory with varying clinical presentations. Despite the radiation dose, we prefer CT as the initial procedure because of its ability to consistently visualize the entire pancreas and its capability to evaluate adjacent nodes. Others may prefer ultrasound, resorting to CT if the diagnosis is not made by that modality. The age groups of these patients makes the radiation risk negligible. Figure 7–7 shows our approach to suspected pancreatic mass. The radiation dose of alternate methods of radiologic procedures is shown on Table 7–3.

Liver

There are many techniques capable of imaging the liver. Since the technecium sulfur colloid scan is very sensitive, easy to perform and provides valuable functional information, we prefer this as the initial procedure in detecting focal liver masses. The nuclear medicine scan, however, is relatively nonspecific and unless a positive finding can be correlated with clin-

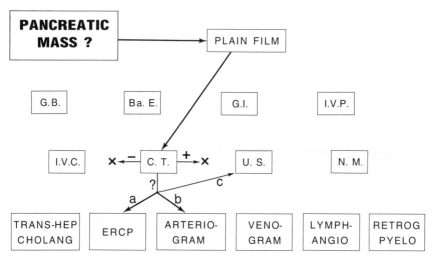

a = Borderline size.   b = Vascular tumor < 2cm.   c = Motion artifact.

Fig 7–7.—Diagnostic approach to suspected pancreatic masses. CT is initial primary procedure, bypassing once-routine barium studies (Ba.E., G.I.). If CT is unequivocally positive or negative, further diagnostic imaging is generally not necessary. Otherwise, it is important to use other procedures after CT. Endoscopic retrograde cholangiopancreatography (ERCP) may be valuable after negative or equivocal CT and in conjunction with a strong clinical suspicion. Angiography is performed routinely for suspected islet cell tumors after negative CT. Sonography is useful in very thin patients or where there is a motion artifact in the CT study.

ical presentation, it often must be complemented by CT or ultrasound. Occasionally, a negative isotopic scan is followed by a positive CT or ultrasound done because the clinical suspicion "outweighs" the negative isotopic scan. This is relatively rare, since the nuclear medicine scan is extremely sensitive but not very specific. See Fig 7–8 and Table 7–4 for the radiation dose with various combinations of diagnostic procedures.

Obstructive Jaundice

The radiologic challenge is to separate jaundice with and without dilated ducts. Although occasionally obstructive jaundice can occur with nondilated ducts, as in sclerosing cholangitis, dilatation usually means obstruction. Ultrasound is a procedure easily performed without ionizing radiation and is highly accurate in detecting dilated from nondilated ducts. Although with ultrasound the cause of obstruction may frequently be identified, other procedures may be required to identify the cause or site of obstruction for the appropriate treatment. IV cholangiography has been largely

TABLE 7–3.—PANCREATIC MASS*

	DOSE
a) CT	10 Rads
b) CT, ERCP	36 Rads
c) CT, Art.	74 Rads
d) CT, US	10 Rads
e) BaE, GI, IVP, IVC	54 Rads
f) CT, US, Art., ERCP, BaE, GI, IVP, IVC	155 Rads

*See Fig 7–1 for legend and caveat.

replaced by ultrasound, since it is unlikely to visualize the common duct where the bilirubin is above 4 mgm/dl. Even when the bilirubin is only minimally elevated, the clinician may still elect to perform ultrasound because of the risk of reaction of the contrast agent and the radiation dose. Our recommended approach is shown in Figure 7–9.

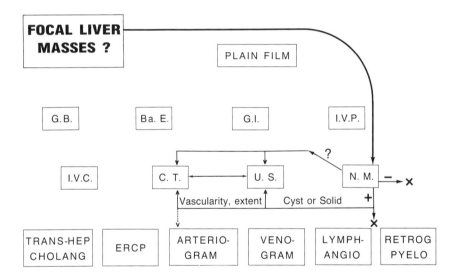

X = STOP

Fig 7–8.—Diagnostic approach for focal liver masses. Radionuclide colloid scan (N.M.) is initial procedure of choice. Diagnostic workup may end with unequivocally positive or negative radioisotopic scan. Utrasound and CT are useful supplementary tests to differentiate cystic from solid focal lesions (sonography), to assess vascularity and extent of disease, or for equivocal and selected negative radionuclide scans. Angiography is recommended routinely when hepatic resection is planned to demonstrate vascular supply and in selected cases (e.g., hemangiomas).

TABLE 7–4.—FOCAL LIVER MASS*

	DOSE
N.M.	1 Rad†
N.M., US	1 Rad†
N.M., US, CT	11 Rads†
N.M., US, CT, Art.	75 Rads†

*See legend for Fig 7–1 and caveat.
†Includes whole-body dose contribution.

Gallbladder

The correct diagnosis of gallbladder disease is extremely important since cholecystitis is the most frequent cause of surgery in the adult and a common cause of hospitalization.

It is useful to separate gallbladder disease into acute and chronic. The presentation of right upper quadrant pain is a differential diagnosis of gallbladder disease and inflammation, or even tumor, of adjacent organs (e.g., head of pancreas, right kidney, liver). We then prefer ultrasound as the initial procedure since it can evaluate all of the organs which may be responsible for the symptoms.

When gallstones are suspected in a nonacute setting, the oral cholecystogram is a reliable procedure, easily performed and which yields functional information. The radiation dose is balanced, in part, by the age of the patient with this disease. This approach is illustrated in Figures 7–10 and 7–11. The dose of radiation with correlation of these various procedures is shown in Table 7–5.

Metastatic Bone Disease

The most sensitive screening examination for the majority of skeletal metastases, particularly in the asymptomatic stage, is the ^{99m}Tc-labeled phosphate bone scan (N.M.). Its detection rate approaches 100% in metastases from lung, prostate, breast and lymphoma. Increased activity occurs due to local increased blood flow on incorporation of the isotope into bone. It

TABLE 7–5.—GALLBLADDER DISEASE*

	DOSE
a) GB	5 Rads
b) GB, US	5 Rads
c) GB, US, IVC	21 Rads
d) GB, US, N.M.	6 Rads†
e) N.M.	1 Rad†

*See legend for Fig 7–1 and caveat.
†Includes whole-body contribution.

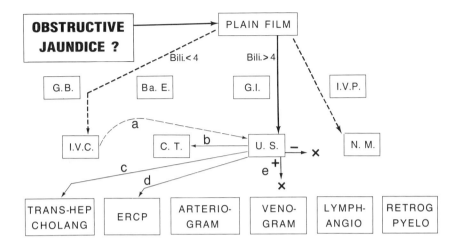

a = Nonvisual.   b = Cause not apparent.   c = With proximal obst.

d = With distal obst.   e = Obstructing mass visualized.   ✗ = STOP

Fig 7–9.—Diagnostic approach for obstructive jaundice. Sonography is the initial imaging procedure if serum bilirubin precludes successful performance of intravenous cholangiography. If ultrasound is negative, bile duct obstruction can be excluded, except in rare cases such as sclerosing cholangitis (see text). If ultrasound demonstrates common bile duct obstruction and its causes **(e),** no further imaging studies are necessary. Otherwise, CT may be performed to demonstrate distal obstructing mass **(b);** transhepatic cholangiography is indicated for proximal obstructing lesions **(c);** and endoscopic retrograde cholangiopancreatography (ERCP) may be necessary if distal obstructing lesion is not apparent with other imaging methods **(d).** Because partially-obstructing common duct stones can be missed by ultrasound, intravenous cholangiography (I.V.C.) has been recommended for mildly jaundiced patients *(dashed arrows).* It is to be followed by ultrasound if there is no cholangiographic visualization **(a).** In practice, most referring physicians have revised this latter pathway. Newer hepatobiliary radioisotopes (N.M.) that have been reliable even in moderately jaundiced patients *(dotted arrow)* may become either the initial imaging procedure, expecially where sonography is not established, or a valuable supplementary procedure, for example, as in biliary obstruction due to sclerosing cholangitis or extensive metastasis.

is frequently positive in the absence of radiographically demonstrated lesions. This procedure will give false negative results, however, in certain tumor types where increased vascularity does not occur, or where osteoblastic activity is not increased, such as in multiple myeloma. Negative bone scans in myeloma may be seen in up to 50% of radiographically demonstrated lesions.

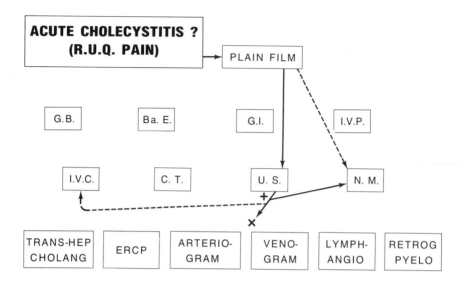

Fig 7–10.—Diagnostic approach to right upper quadrant pain with suspected acute cholecystitis. Sonography is performed after a plain film because of its capability to demonstrate not only the gallbladder, but also pathologic changes in adjacent organs that may mimic acute cholecystitis. Unless there is a large impacted stone, cystic duct obstruction cannot be established by ultrasound. For this purpose, radionuclide hepatobiliary scan (N.M.) or, if not available, intravenous cholangiography (I.V.C.) is indicated *(dashed arrow)*. Where information about adjacent organs is not desirable, radionuclide method becomes first procedure in acute cholecystitis *(dotted arrow)*.

Because of its sensitivity, the radionuclide scan (N.M.) should be the first procedure performed in the search for skeletal metastatic disease with very few exceptions. This may be all that is needed if the patient's symptoms, the appearance and location of the scan, and the patient's known tumor fits. If the scan is positive in an asymptomatic area or if the scan abnormality could be produced by a benign process, then plain radiographs may be necessary and even occasionally tomography or CT scanning is required. The latter procedure, in addition to identifying a lesion, is of particular help in establishing the extent of disease for radiation therapy ports, especially if in a complex bone and if it is important to know the soft tissue extension of the tumor for radiation therapy. In general, however, the latter two procedures are not frequently required. Figure 7–12 is a diagram that illustrates this approach. The radiologic exposure of these procedures can be found in Table 7–6.

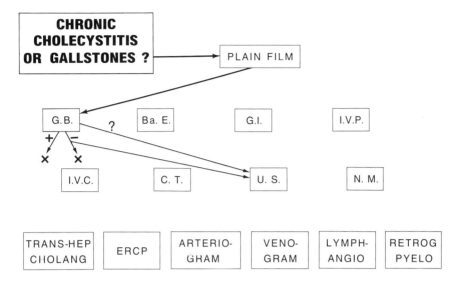

Fig 7–11.—Diagnostic approach to chronic cholecystitis or cholelithiasis. Oral cholecystogram (G.B.) after a plain film is the choice. Sonography is a valuable supplementary test if there is suboptimal or nonvisualization on oral cholecystography, or if strong clinical suspicion of gallstones persists despite negative oral cholecystogram. In pregnancy and renal failure, sonography has been performed as initial procedure.

Hypertension

The standard IVP and variations of its routine performance are still recommended by many authors as an early screening procedure in clinically selected cases of hypertension.[61, 62] Despite its limitations in identifying a

TABLE 7–6.—SKELETAL METASTASIS*

	DOSE
a) N.M.	1 Rad†
b) Met. Survey	10 Rads†
c) N.M., plain films (2)	3 Rads†
d) N.M., plain films (2), Tomo.‡	13 Rads†
e) N.M., plain films (2), Tomo., CT	23 Rads†
f) N.M., plain films (2), CT	13 Rads†
g) Met. Survey, Tomo., CT	30 Rads
i) Met. Survey, CT	20 Rads

*See Fig 7–1 for legend and caveat.
†Includes whole body dose component.
‡Tomo = Conventional Tomography.

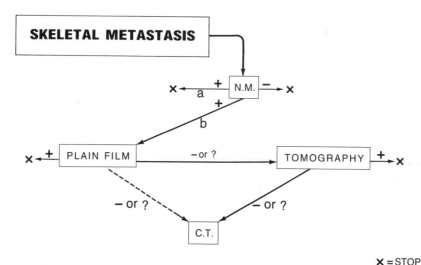

a = If scan fits clinically and is diagnostic.

b = If scan could be from benign disease or asymptomatic done for staging.

Fig 7–12.—Diagnostic approach for suspected skeletal metastasis. (See text for explanation.) If the primary lesion is suspected to be multiple myeloma, the N.M. scan is excluded and a radiographic metastatic survey is carried out.

renovascular cause of hypertension, they point to the simplicity of its performance, wide availability and a high lay and professional acceptance. Further, it may aid in detecting other causes of hypertension such as tumor, pyelonephritis, polycystic disease or renal infarction.

At The New York Hospital, our approach more recently has been to avoid the IVP in screening hypertension even though it is quite sensitive, since it is relatively nonspecific. It has the disadvantage of a relatively high radiation dose as well as a potential of the reaction to the contrast agent.

We have in many cases, after appropriate clinical and biochemical screening, obtained as the first radiologic procedure—on an outpatient basis—a selective renal vein and inferior vena cava renin collection. With the catheter in place, a digitized intravenous angiogram (DF) can be carried out to visualize the renal arteries.

The initial clinical screening includes a careful history regarding the age, sex, length of time of elevated blood pressure and ease of control. The biochemical screening includes peripheral plasma renin and blood pressure determinations before and after captopril.

If these radiologic studies demonstrate a renal artery cause for the hypertension or if one cannot be excluded, the patient is admitted for aortic catheterization and a selective renal arteriogram. A transluminal angioplasty is then performed at the same sitting if a stenotic segment is identified.[63] This approach is described in the flow chart in Figure 7–13.

Intra-abdominal Abscesses

The morbidity and mortality of intra-abdominal abscesses is directly in proportion to the time it takes to make the diagnosis, localize it and initiate appropriate therapy.

The etiologies of intra-abdominal abscesses have vastly changed in recent years. Appendicitis in the past accounted for up to 50% of cases, while now surgery and trauma are the leading causes. The insidious causes of abscesses are increasing in number and therefore are often overlooked. These are associated with drug abuse, chemotherapy, steroids and immunosuppression. The selection of the proper, or proper sequence, of radiologic procedures is dictated by the clinical suspicion of its cause. This obviously reflects a careful history and physical examination, evaluation of pertinent laboratory findings and clinical judgment.

The anatomic site also varies the clinical presentation: the retroperitoneum often presents with minimal symptoms; the peritoneal cavity with

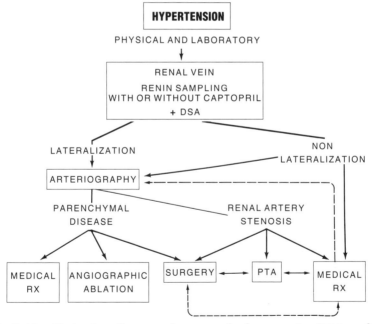

Fig 7–13.—Evaluation of suspected renovascular hypertension (DSA = digital subtraction angiography; PTA = percutaneous transluminal angioplasty).

symptoms. Age may minimize symptomatology, even though peritoneal in origin.

The morphologic appearance and the ease of radiologically diagnosing or imaging an abscess, depends on the stage of its formation. When only a phlegmon is present, only altered organ contours and obliterated adjacent soft tissue planes will be observed. As organization occurs, the collection becomes solid. With further maturation, the center becomes liquified; and finally necrotic debris develops in the center.

The three modalities which are useful in the diagnosis are ultrasound, CT and nuclear medicine:

The *ultrasound* examination has a reported "high" accuracy rate. Its accuracy however is subject to variation depending on the skill of the examiner. It is most useful in the right upper quadrant and in the pelvis, where the organs in those areas lend themselves to ultrasonic imaging.

The *CT* examination gives the best anatomic information and is helpful in guiding percutaneous culturing and drainage of the abscess. The CT appearance will vary depending on the stage of the abscess: (1) When only phlegmon is present, there is only loss of definition of adjacent organs. (2) As a solid abscess forms, a soft tissue mass of low density appears. (3) As the abscess becomes necrotic, its density increases. At this stage it may be difficult to separate the abscess from neoplasm.

There are two types of *radionuclide scans* used in diagnosing an abscess.[64] Those that accumulate in normal parenchyma with the abscess producing a filling defect in the organ (^{99m}Tc-sulfur colloid) and those that accumulate at the site of inflammation (^{67}Ga citrate and In-wbc). The ^{99m}Tc-sulfur colloid scan is useful in the diagnosis of suspected intrahepatic or intrasplenic collections where diseases appear as filling defects in the outlined organ.

The advantage of gallium scanning is that it examines the entire abdomen. It is, however, more accurate and is positive earlier with large mature abscesses. It may miss early phlegmon. The disadvantages of gallium scanning are a high false positive accumulation in normal structures, such as the colon, and the fact that it may require up to 72 hours to make a diagnosis. There is also overlap with certain neoplasms such as lymphomas.

The radiologic approach to the diagnosis of intra-abdominal abscesses will vary depending on the clinical presentation. Our recommended approach at The New York Hospital varies between those patients presenting with a fever of undetermined origin and those with some localized findings or a clinical suspicion of organ involvement giving localizing clues.

The CT scan is recommended as the first procedure with fever and no localizing clues. It not only is highly accurate in the diagnosis, but also the most useful in the localization for either percutaneous or surgical drainage.

If the CT is negative and biliary tract disease is not excluded, an ultrasound examination is profitable. Further, if a definable abscess is not present on CT and phlegmon is clinically suspected, a gallium scan may be performed, but as stated above its accuracy is decreased with this type of pathology. When the CT examination is positive and there is question of the collection being noninfected, a gallium scan may be helpful (Fig 7–14).

If a specific location is suspected CT may not be the first procedure performed. If localizing signs point to the right upper quadrant, an ultrasound examination is usually done. Ultrasound also examines the pelvis and adnexa as well. If osteomyelitis is the suspected diagnosis, the nuclear medicine bone scan is done first. CT, however, is clearly superior in the retroperitoneum, the left upper quadrant and bowel-related pelvic abscesses. This approach is illustrated in Figure 7–15. The dose from these procedures or combination of procedures is shown in Table 7–7.

UTILIZATION

Many articles have been written alluding to the overutilization of x-rays. Undue dependence on x-ray rather than clinical observation, lack of proper screening by the radiologist, patient demand, reimbursement policies, in-

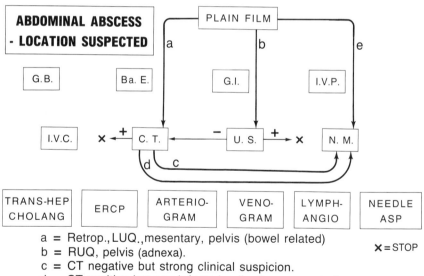

a = Retrop., LUQ., mesentary, pelvis (bowel related)
b = RUQ, pelvis (adnexa).
c = CT negative but strong clinical suspicion.
d = CT positive but non-infected collection suspected.
e = Osteomyelitis suspected after recent trauma or surgery.

✗ = STOP

Fig 7–14.—Diagnostic approach to the detection of an intra-abdominal abscess if there are no clinical clues as to origin.

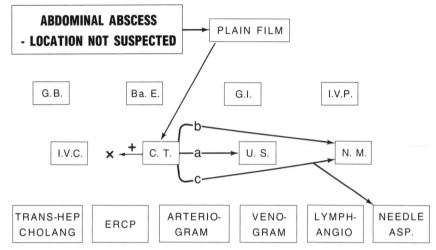

a = Gallbladder, billary tree.   **✗** = STOP
b = CT negative but strong clinical suspicion.
c = CT positive but non-infected collection suspected.

Fig 7–15.—Diagnostic approach to the detection of an intra-abdominal abscess would depend on the suspected location.

stitutional requirements and preventive and defensive medicine are but a few of the causes.[65–67]

Radiologic procedures are performed either because the patient is symptomatic or has a known disease and is being followed. The examination potentially has the capability of acquiring information for management or as a screening procedure to diagnose asymptomic disease. Many procedures continue to be performed despite evidence that demonstrates their worthlessness.

TABLE 7–7.—ABDOMINAL ABSCESS*

	DOSE
a. CT	10 Rads
b. CT, US	10 Rads
c. CT, NM	11 Rads†
d. CT, Needle Asp.	30/10 Rads‡

*See Fig 7–1 for legend and caveat.
†Includes whole body dose contribution.
‡The dose is 30 rads if the aspiration is done under fluoroscopic control; it will be 10 rads if it is performed under ultrasonic control.

Pelvimetry

Pelvimetry frequently can be avoided by the use of ultrasound.[68, 69] Since this examination represents the greatest source of fetal irradiation, careful selection of patients should be carried out. Careful clinical evaluation, review of films obtained prior to pregnancy, and, as stated, ultrasound many times can preclude the need for pelvimetry. It is generally accepted that the induction of labor, breech presentation or "youth" are not of themselves indication for pelvimetry. BRH has published a document[58] that discusses the utilization of pelvimetry and includes the following statement developed by an expert physician panel which may become a guide for the use of pelvimetry:

"Pelvimetry is not usually necessary or helpful in making the decision to perform a cesarean section. Therefore, pelvimetry should be performed only when the physician caring for the patient feels that pelvimetry will contribute to the decisions concerning diagnosis or treatment. In those few instances, the reason for requesting the pelvimetry should be written on the patient's chart. This statement does not apply to x-ray examinations for purposes other than measurement of the pelvis."

Skull X-Rays

TRAUMA.—Several studies have conclusively shown an overutilization of plain skull x-rays following trauma, both in adults and children.[59, 70, 71] Overutilization is demonstrated by the low incidence of skull fracture with insignificant trauma and lack of correlation between skull fracture and cerebral injury. At our institution in many instances, CT scanning has replaced the plain skull x-rays when significant head trauma has occurred.

HEADACHE.—Clinical selection for the radiologic workup of headache is most important since every headache cannot undergo a radiologic workup. Headaches are estimated to effect 90% of the population resulting in 16,000,000 visits to physicians every year. Compare this to 6,300 persons who die yearly from brain tumors.[71] The causes of headache are both intracranial and extracranial and proper clinical screening not only eliminates the need for medical imaging, but the selection of the examination (i.e., sinus, brain CT, cervical spine, etc.).

Plain radiographs are often improperly utilized to attempt to diagnose the external and intracranial causes of headaches (e.g., sinusitis, cervical arthritis, brain tumors, etc.). They rarely demonstrate intracranial abnormality with the occasional exception of hyperostosis associated with meningioma, occasional calcified neoplasm, abnormalities of the sella seen in either primary pituitary lesion, or in chronic elevated increased intracranial pressure. In most instances when extracranial pathology is excluded as the etiology of headaches, skull films should be omitted and CT performed directly.

Though the cost of a CT examination is relatively high, the quality of information acquired is also high. The radiation dose is modest in proportion to its yield of diagnostic information. Often a specific diagnosis can be made without any additional radiologic procedures or laboratory tests. It is necessary, however, in certain clinical situations, to supplement CT by angiography and, rarely, by pneumoencephalography.

For the last 20 years the nuclear medicine scan has been an excellent screening method for intracranial causes of headache. It has largely been replaced by CT scanning. The lack of specificity of the N.M. scan and the additional information available on the CT scan (ventricle size, characteristic of mass, etc.) has been largely responsible for this. Occasionally, however, the nuclear medicine (NM) scan may be positive with a negative CT scan in cases of subacute to chronic meningitis or in early brain abscesses.

The arteriogram is now mainly used in diagnosing intrinsic lesions of the cerebral vascular system, CT replacing its priority role of evaluating brain parenchyma, ventricles and cisterns. An arteriogram usually follows a positive CT scan to define the blood supply to a tumor already diagnosed. The exception may be if the headache has an abrupt onset, stiff neck and blood in the cerebrospinal fluid. A suspected aneurysm may be diagnosed or excluded by an arteriogram. The CT exam however may add information such as the extent of hematoma and ventricular size and often may be the primary procedure.

The pneumoencephalogram, with the current availability of modern CT scanning, is rarely carried out. Its associated discomfort, radiation dose and morbidity makes its use limited. It may, however, be required in suspected brain stem masses or masses of the posterior fossa. NMR may soon remove even this indication for pneumoencephalography due to its ability to image through bone.

In general, if a headache is clinically thought to be of sinus origin, plain sinus radiographs should be obtained. If the clinical situation suggests a subarachnoid bleed, an arteriogram may be done. The vast majority of times, however, if good clinical screening suggests a tumor as the cause of headache, the CT scan is the initial procedure of choice.

Barium Enema

The overutilization of barium enemas has been stressed by MacEwan.[72] In his study, the most justified indication for this exam is suspicion of carcinoma. There was a high positive correlation between strong suspicion of carcinoma and the radiologic findings. When the clinician thought with a high degree of certainty that the exam would be positive, it was in a great number of cases; when the index of suspicion was low, so was the incidence of pathology. In the pediatric age group, high return was experienced with such indications as intusseception, colitis and Hirschstring's disease, but low return was experienced with such indications as abdominal pain, constipation, and blood loss. MacEwan's conclusion was that good clinical judgment was the best indication for selection of a barium enema.

Mammography

Much controversy exists concerning the performance of mammography. Some concern exists over the possibility that the radiation used in the examination may, in some cases, induce more carcinoma than is detected by the technique. Because the exact risk of radiation-induced breast carcinoma is unknown, mammography is therefore controversial.

It has been determined by the first large scale breast cancer screening programs that mammography coupled with physical examination decreases breast cancer mortality in women over the age of 50[73] by detecting cancer in the preclinical stage.

The benefit of mammography in early detection as it affects survival or cure justifies its proper use. As in all cases, however, clinical judgment should dictate mammography's role in each clinical situation. Needless mammography in low risk patients, patients on whom the exam has little hope of demonstrating cancer (young, fibrous breasts) is to be avoided but patients in whom the benefit clearly outweighs the risks, (e.g., over 50, strong familial history), should not be deprived of the benefits of mammography.

At the time of this writing a committee of the American College of Radiology has published a current version of the guidelines for mammography which are a slight modification of their recommendations in 1976. A brief summary of this is taken from the ACR Bulletin, November, 1982.[74]

"Mammography is an essential part of the evaluation of the patient and when optimally combined with physical examination, offers a high degree of accuracy.

Since the incidence of naturally occurring breast cancer is considerably higher in symptomatic women, the higher yield of non-palpable cancers results in even greater benefit-risk than in asymptomatic women.

1. These recommendations for periodic screening mammography of women under age 50 are made because of accumulating data on benefits and the lead time gained by earlier detection. The American College of Radiology believes that these recommendations represent the most prudent advice based upon the best currently available evidence.
2. All women should be taught proper breast self-examination by age 20 and should have an annual examination of the breast after age 35.
3. The first, or baseline, mammograms should be obtained by age 40. An earlier age is preferable when there is a personal history of pre-menopausal breast cancer or a history of pre-menopausal breast cancer in the patient's mother and/or sisters.
4. Subsequent mammographic examination should be performed at one to two

year intervals determined by the combined analysis of physical and mammographic findings and other risk factors, unless medically indicated sooner.

5. Annual mammography and physical examination are recommended for all women over age 50."

The policy at The New York Hospital has been that mammography is performed on patients with significant symptoms and signs at any age. Specifically, if a lump is felt, the exam may diagnose it as malignant or benign. Evaluation of the opposite breast should also be carried out, if the mass appears malignant since there is a 3 to 5% evidence of simultaneous bilateral cancer. Pain and nipple discharge also are evaluated by mammography. In asymptomatic patients, any patient with a previous mastectomy has mammography done since there is a 17% incidence of carcinoma in the second breast. In addition, if the patient has large and lumpy breasts mammography may have to be done, since palpation is difficult. If an unknown primary tumor is being sought with metastasis compatible with those from a breast tumor or if an axillary lymph node is felt, mammography is done.

Finally, if a strong familial history of breast carcinoma exists (i.e., mother, sister) a screening mammogram is recommended to be done some time between the ages of 35 and 40. Without strong family history, a routine mammogram is obtained between ages 40 and 45. The subsequent frequency of screening is at least once every 3 years; in the high risk group at least once every 2 years. In general, the frequency should increase with age and susceptibility.

Chest X-Ray

The radiation dose of the chest x-ray when properly performed is extremely low. There is minimal bone marrow dose and essentially no gonadal dose. It is therefore important to obtain a chest x-ray on any patient who is symptomatic or when history or physical findings suggest the possibility of chest disease. Further, in selected asymptomatic populations shown to have a high incidence of chest disease (i.e., smokers) regular chest examination should be performed.

The diagnosis of early lung cancer is extremely important because only Stage I lung cancer is routinely curable by surgical methods. Stages II and III lung cancer are only rarely associated with long-term survival. For this reason, radiographic screening programs for detection of early (Stage I) lung cancer have been attempted.

In the past, x-ray screening programs have not proved effective for a variety of reasons: poor quality films, single reading of radiographs, use of reduced format radiographs or photofluorograms, low kVp technique and lack of availability of previous comparison radiographs. Early diagnosis of lung cancer by means of screening radiography has been markedly improved in three National Cancer Institute screening programs; at the National Lung Program sponsored by Memorial Sloan-Kettering Cancer Center, the Johns Hopkins Lung Project and the Mayo Lung Project. The improvement in radiographic diagnosis has resulted from independent double reading of radiographs with a system of arbitration involving evaluation by a third radiologist, use of PA and lateral full size 14" × 17" films, high kVp technique (140 kVp) and comparison with prior radiographs that are kept on file.[75]

Yearly radiographic screening of 10,000 high-risk male cigarette smokers at the National Lung Program in New York City has proved effective in diagnosing 40% of all lung cancers at Stage I. Small cell lung cancer has not proved amenable to early x-ray diagnosis, but the results with epidermoid and adenocarcinoma are encouraging, with frequent diagnosis of those latter histologic types at Stage I, when they most often present as small (usually) peripheral lung nodules.[76] The long-term disease free survival in this group of patients has been excellent.[77]

In a recent ACR bulletin[78] the referral criteria developed by a BRH-sponsored physician panel for routine screening chest x-ray examination were stated as follows:

"Referral Criteria for Routine Screening Chest X-Ray Examinations
  I. Referral Criteria for Mandated Routine Screening Chest X-Ray Examinations
      There are a variety of instances where free-standing screening chest x-ray examinations are performed in asymptomatic persons solely by administrative mandate or protocol. This practice is based on the assumption that significant disease can be detected in a silent phase when it is more amenable to successful medical treatment. The productivity of such mandated chest examinations in random populations is therefore dependent on the prevalence of existing disease in asymptomatic persons and whether its early detection does in fact effect a significant reduction in morbidity and mortality.
      The yield of unsuspected disease (e.g., lung cancer, heart disease and tuberculosis) found by routine mandated screening chest x-ray examinations of unselected populations, not based on history, physical examination, or specific diagnostic testing has been shown to be of insufficient clinical value to justify the monetary cost, added radiation exposure and subject inconvenience of the examination.
      It is therefore recommended that all such mandated routine screening examinations of unselected populations be discontinued, unless a significant yield can be shown.
      This statement does not preclude chest x-ray examinations based on individual history, physical examination, or specific diagnostic testing (e.g., sputum cytology, electrocardiography, and skin test); or in selected populations shown to have significant yields of previously undiagnosed disease.
 II. *Referral Criteria for Routine Prenatal Chest X-Ray Examinations*
      The yield of unsuspected disease found by routine chest x-ray examination of unselected pregnant patients (i.e., by protocol or by mandate) has been

shown to be of insufficient clinical value to justify the radiation exposure, inconvenience to the pregnant patient, and monetary cost.

It is therefore recommended that all such routine prenatal chest x-ray examinations be discontinued.

This statement does not preclude prenatal chest x-ray examinations based on individual history, physical examination, or specific diagnostic testing, or in selected populations shown to have significant yields of previously undiagnosed disease.

III. *Referral Criteria for Routine Hospital Admission Chest X-Ray Examinations*

The rationale for obtaining routine chest radiographs of patients admitted to hospitals is to discover unsuspected disease which might directly threaten the health of the patient and/or jeopardize the health of those coming in contact with the patient. However, available evidence suggests that the yield of clinically significant information (not available from history, physical examination, or previous diagnostic testing) from such routine screening chest radiographs is low.

It is therefore recommended that routine chest radiographs not be required solely because of hospital admission.

This recommendation should not be construed as precluding or advising against the ordering of chest x-ray examinations (1) on the basis of history, physical examination, or specific diagnostic testing, or (2) in selected patient populations in which a significant yield has been previously substantiated or is considered highly likely pending appropriate substantiation.

IV. *Chest X-Ray Examinations in Occupational Medicine*
Preemployment/Preplacement Examinations for Appropriate Job Placement

Preplacement chest x-ray examinations should be done selectively based on pertinent factors in the (1) occupational and medical history, (2) clinical examination, and (3) proposed work assignment.

Job Exposure Surveillance

Chest x-ray surveillance of persons who work with or may be exposed to substances that adversely affect pulmonary function or cause pulmonary disease should be based on a periodicity consistent with the current understanding of the disease process.

Periodic Examination Unrelated to Job Exposure

The yield of unsuspected disease (e.g., lung cancer, heart disease, and tuberculosis) found by periodic chest x-ray examinations of unselected populations, not based on history, physical examination, or specific diagnostic testing has been shown to be of insufficient clinical value to justify the monetary cost, added radiation exposure, and subject inconvenience of the examination. It is therefore recommended that such routine examinations be discontinued.

This statement does not preclude chest x-ray examinations based on individual history, physical examination, or specific diagnostic testing (e.g., sputum cytology, electrocardiography, and skin test); or in selected populations shown to have significant yields of previously undiagnosed disease.

V. *Chest X-Ray Examinations for Tuberculosis Detection and Control*

A chest x-ray examination should always be obtained whenever a specific medical indication exists (e.g., relevant history, symptoms, and/or significant tuberculin skin test reaction). However, there are several situations where x-ray examinations have traditionally been performed solely because of administrative mandate, protocol, or by routine. The yield of tuberculosis cases found by screening or repeated chest x-ray examinations has not been shown to be of sufficient clinical value or productivity to justify the inconvenience to the subject, monetary costs, or added radiation exposure.

Chest X-Ray Examinations for Employment

Mandated chest x-ray examinations as a condition of initial or continuing employment have not been shown to be of sufficient productivity to justify their continued use for tuberculosis detection.

Chest X-Ray Examinations in Long-Term Care Facilities

Because conventional tuberculin skin testing may not be a reliable screening method in older and/or chronically ill persons and because these individuals may be at high risk of having tuberculosis, the results of recent examination should be obtained by the nursing home. Only if unavailable, a chest x-ray examination should be performed on admission. In the absence of clinical symptoms, repeated chest x-ray examinations have not shown to be of sufficient clinical value or productivity to justify their continued use.

Repeated Chest X-Ray Examination of Tuberculin Reactors

After an initial evaluation, which should include a chest x-ray examination, repeated chest x-ray examinations of individuals with significant tuberculin reactions (without current disease), whether or not they have been treated with isoniazid, have not been shown to be of sufficient clinical value or productivity to justify their continued use.

Routine Follow-up of Tuberculosis Patients Who Have Completed Treatment

Repeated chest x-ray examinations of asymptomatic tuberculosis patients who have completed treatment have been shown to be of insufficient clinical value or productivity to justify their continued use.

Routine Periodic Chest X-Ray Examination During Tuberculosis Treatment

Radiographic stability does not indicate success or failure of chemotherapy as reliably as the results of sputum smear and culture, and assessment of symptoms and clinical status. However, an occasional x-ray examination may have value in confirming bacteriologic and clinical findings and enhancing patient compliance."

These recommendations, based on radiation dosage, patient inconvenience and cost, are that screening examinations in unselected population yield insufficient information in the situations they discuss. They do not preclude their use, however, based on history, physical examinations, specific diagnostic testing such as skin tests, electrocardiography or sputum cytology.

Though the authors agree in principle with these conclusions, we would like to emphasize that a properly performed chest x-ray with attention to dose reduction, image quality and interpretation gives the patient an examination with minimal radiation dose and maximum information. Since cost and patient convenience are real considerations, other procedures in medicine must be examined under the same criteria. For example, an annual physical examination in certain age groups may be of low yield as are many routine laboratory determinations. The return of a properly performed chest x-ray may well be among the most effective examinations considering cost, risk and benefit.

Finally, a baseline chest x-ray in most instances should be obtained which will greatly aid in evaluating a subsequent chest x-ray, at a time when the patient is symptomatic.

Nuclear Magnetic Resonance Clinical Application

At the time of this writing, NMR is evolving as an important diagnostic tool.[79] As pointed out, primarily it does not involve potentially harmful ionizing radiation. Further safety advantages are that since contrast agents are not used, there is no risk of anaphylactic reaction. Because of its ability to measure flow it may also replace some arteriography obviating the risks of that procedure.

It has advantages over other imaging modalities in that the images produced are not only based on "density differences" and can, for example, separate a blood filled vessel from an adjacent tumor.

It would appear at this time that clearly NMR will become the procedure of choice in the diagnosis of many clinical problems. This appears most promising in the following: (1) The diagnosis of pituitary tumors. The CT scan is impeded by bony density of the splenoid bone. (2) The posterior fossa and brain. The CT scan is impeded by the bony density of the occipital bone and upper cervical spine. (3) Multiple sclerosis. (4) Disc disease. This spinal cord and disc is directly visualized, rather than depending on the indirect evidence of a myelogram. (5) Hydrocephalus of the newborn and the pediatrics age group. The resolution will equal or exceed that of ultrasound and CT without the risks of CT (i.e., contrast injection and ionizing radiation). (6) Evaluation of tumors of the thorax. The limitation of CT scanning has been separating vascular structure from solid tumors without knowing detailed knowledge of the anatomy of the thorax. The image as seen with NMR is completely different from that of adjacent normal vascular structures. (7) Evaluation of large vessel disease (aneurysm and stenosis). (8) Evaluation of transplanted and failing kidney.

It is also clear that there will be many more applications after evaluation and experience. Among these are certain to be evaluation of cardiac disease in both adults and children, tumor detection, bone and joint disease, and inflammatory processes.

PREGNANCY AND RADIATION

Examination of a woman of childbearing age requires special consideration and is difficult to summarize without specific clinical information. The time of the menstrual cycle, the stage of pregnancy, the dose of radiation and the time over which the radiation is received become significant factors. Despite many studies (both on experimental animals and extrapolated human experience) it is still not known what dose is harmful.

It is not an uncommon occurrence that after a radiologic examination, the patient discovers that she was pregnant at the time and she and her physician become concerned. Termination of the pregnancy is often considered. To make this decision, some estimates of the risk must be given by the physician. It would, however, be extremely unlikely for a patient undergoing a diagnostic examination to receive a dose which might indicate the desirability of an abortion.

This advice must be given in relation to nonradiologic risks, i.e., from 4 to 6% of births have varying degrees of congenital defects regardless of radiation history. The increased risk of congenital defect below a 10 rad exposure to the fetus at any stage of pregnancy is minimal when compared to this figure.[41, 45]

Several other facts, however, should be considered; greatest vulnerability to the fetus is the 10th day through the 10th week after conception; the risk is probably negligible at 5 rads or less when compared to the other risks of pregnancy; the risk of malformation is significantly increased when the radiation dose is above 15 rads. There is no measurable advantage in scheduling diagnostic x-ray examinations at any particular time during a normal cycle.[80–82] The developing ovum is at risk prior to ovulation as well as after. We do not therefore see any advantage to the scheduling of elective radiographic procedures relative to a patient's menstrual status. The possibility of an early pregnancy should be discussed with the patient. Where medically appropriate, consideration should be given to minimizing potential fetal irradiation by limiting the scope of the examination. Fetal irradiation can also be reduced by technical means, such as shielding and collimation, which can be used during the performance of a necessary examination.

One might conclude then that a fetal exposure of 20 rads at 3 weeks post conception might suggest consideration of a therapeutic abortion. A dose of 5 rads at 20 weeks would probably not suggest an abortion. The cases in between can only depend on judgment and must include patient input with factors such as estimate of the "odds" (based on the dose and time of pregnancy), religious background and the patient's and family's psychologic response to the pregnancy. For a more detailed discussion, the reader is referred to Report No. 54 of the National Council on Radiation Protection and Measurements (NCRP).[81, 82]

The risk of fetal cancer induction has been discussed in Chapter 5, Section 3.

8 / Evaluation of Radiation Risk

RADIATION RISK TO THE ADULT PATIENT

THE TWO PRINICIPAL RISKS OF IRRADIATION at diagnostic imaging levels are the induction of cancer and the production of heritable mutations. Both of these are low probability stochastic risks. The vast majority of patients will suffer no injury whatsoever as a consequence of the imaging procedure. A minute fraction of irradiated patients will incur radiation damage as a consequence of their examinations. However, only a fraction of even these patients will ever express their radiation injury.

For public health purposes, one usually takes a very conservative approach to estimating the radiation risk from an exposure. Therefore a zero threshold, linear, no repair model is customarily used to relate dose to risk. This model gives an upper limit to the risk associated with low doses of radiation. We can combine this model with the BRH measurements reported in XES-70 and reach an upper limit on the present radiologic risk from diagnostic radiology. This upper limit of risk together with typical organ dose data from XES-70[14, 83] are used for the estimates presented in Table 8–1. The reader should note that this procedure combines a conservative dose effect model with a probable overestimate of the dose delivered by specific examinations in the mid 1980s. *Thus, the radiation risks predicted from this combination of factors are worst case estimates and may be in fact more than several times the true risks.*

We have estimated the leukemia (and bone cancer) risk associated with each of the examinations on our list of examinations by taking an age weighted linear risk estimate of 2.24 radiogenic leukemias per rad per million persons per year (BEIR III, p. 204) and by assuming that this risk is constant for twenty-five years after a ten year latent period. Thus the lifetime risk per rad (without adjusting for intervening mortality) is about 56 fatalities per million. It is to be noted that the number of expressed radiogenic injuries must be less than the tabulated values due to the age distribution of the irradiated population. The BEIR Committee has calculated a lifetime risk, weighted according to life tables (on a per million basis), of 56.6 leukemias per rad for males and 38.4 for females. A sample calculation follows: The average marrow dose for a lumbar spine examination is 347 millirads (0.347 rad). This is multiplied by the lifetime risk of a one rad

TABLE 8–1.—PROBABLE MAXIMUM LIFETIME RISKS FROM SELECTED EXAMINATIONS[a]

Examination	AVERAGE MARROW DOSE[b] (MILLIRADS)	FATAL LEUKEMIAS AND BONE CANCERS/MILLION EXAMS[c]	GONADAL DOSE (MILLIRADS) Male	Female	GENETIC DISEASE/ MILLION EXAMS[c]
Spontaneous Incidence		9,800[d]	—[g]	—	107,000[e]
Skull	78	4[f]			—
Chest	10[h]	0.5	—	—	—
Cervical spine	52	3	—	—	—
Thoracic spine	247	10	3	11[f]	6
Lumbar spine	347	20	218	74	400
Intravenous pyelogram	420	20	207	588	300
Gallbladder	168	9	—	78	30
Upper G.I. series	535	30	1[i]	171[i]	70
Barium enema	875	50	175[i]	903[i]	500
K.U.B.	147	8	97	221	100
Pelvis	93	5	364	210	200
Hip	72	4	600	124	300
Dental	9	0.5	—	—	—

[a]Dosimetry from XES-70.
[b]Averaged over total bone marrow in skeleton.
[c]Linear model with full expression of cases produced by radiation.
[d]U.S. lifetime estimates of incidence of leukemia and bone cancer per million (BEIR-III, p. 204).
[e]U.S. current incidence per million live births.
[f]All values have been rounded to one significant figure.
[g]Less than 0.5 millirad per examination.
[h]Photofluorographs are not included.
[i]Radiographic component of examination only.

exposure of 56 cases per million yielding an estimate of 19.4 leukemias (rounded to 20) produced by performing one million lumbar spine examinations.

In like manner, we have estimated the risk of producing a genetic disease by estimating the average doubling dose to be 125 rads (risk per rad = 0.008). The risk of inducing genetic disease as a result of performing a lumbar spine examination may be estimated by taking the male-female average gonadal dose (0.471 rad) and multiplying this value by the risk per rad (0.008) and by the natural incidence (107,000) which yields 402 genetic diseases (rounded to 400) as a result of performing one million lumbar spine examinations on prospective parents. One obvious caution regarding the use of the gonadal dose (and risk) per examination data given here: most radiologic procedures are performed on older patients (i.e., after their children have been born). There is no genetic risk unless the patient becomes a parent after the examination is performed.[83] Thus most radiologic procedures carry no genetic risk.

The large difference between gonadal dose per examination and genetically significant dose per examination (weighted for the probabilities of future children) is shown in Table 8–2. This table does not include further weighting factors for the differences between male and female mutagenic sensitivities. It is interesting to note that the increased ovarian dose found for most procedures will be somewhat ameliorated by the lesser radiosensitivity of the oocyte.

Table 8–1 estimates the probabilities per million examinations of developing radiogenic leukemia and a heritable genetic disease. The risks of inducing other forms of cancer were previously reviewed and included both age and site in estimating the overall risk of radiation. Because of this

TABLE 8–2.—COMPARISON OF GONADAL DOSE AND GENETICALLY SIGNIFICANT DOSE FOR RADIOGRAPHIC EXAMINATIONS ONLY

EXAMINATION	XES-70 GONADAL (MRAD/ EXAMINATION)		GSD* GENETICALLY SIGNIFICANT (MRAD/ EXAMINATION)	
	Male	Female	Male	Female
Upper G.I. series	1	171	—	0.4
Barium enema	175	903	0.3	1.7
Gallbladder		78	—	0.6
IVP	207	588	1.0	2.2
Lumbar spine	218	721	0.5	3.1
Pelvic	364	210	0.7	1.1

*Includes population weighting over age and examination distributions.

complex behavior, and because of the difficulties of assessing organ dose as a general function of the physical variables associated with radiologic imaging, the authors will not attempt to estimate specific organ risks from radiodiagnostic procedures. As a guideline, the solid tumor risk is probably close to the leukemia risk.

Using the absolute risk model, the lifetime radiation risk of being irradiated increases with decreasing age due to the increased time available for expressing any radiation injury in the young. Therefore one tends to avoid routine exposures of younger populations in order to minimize even the small radiologic risk of such exposures. This principle certainly applies to the desire to minimize fetal irradiation.

FERTILITY EFFECTS IN THE ADULT

Stimulation of fertility and transient radiation sterilization occur at acute organ doses above 100 rads. These effects are therefore unimportant in diagnostic imaging. As previously discussed, animal experiments indicate a lessened probability of genetic disease if conception is postponed by a few months after pelvic irradiation at intermediate dose levels.

RISK OF FETAL IRRADIATION

In addition to the risk of cancer induction, the fetus is subject to the additional risk of developmental damage when it is irradiated. The nature of the risk will depend upon the dose and upon the developmental state of the fetus when irradiated. Teratogenic effects appear to have a threshold dose of about 5 to 10 rads.[42] The ovarian doses tabulated in Table 8–1 are a reasonable estimate of the dose received by an early fetus. Thus most single radiologic examinations are below the threshold for developmental defects.

Extensive pelvic radiologic examinations can impose fetal doses exceeding 10 rads and may induce teratogenic effects. Under unusual circumstances, doses in this range may also cause subtle neurologic deficits; the evidence in man is unclear in this respect. The NCRP[81] considers "the risk of fetal irradiation to be negligible at 5 rads or less, when compared to the other risks of pregnancy, and the risk of malformations is significantly increased above control levels only at doses above 15 rads."

9 / Radiation Workers as Patients

MEDICAL RADIATION WORKERS

THE PRACTITIONER MAY HAVE RADIATION WORKERS among his or her patients and may therefore be called upon to give advice regarding the occupational risks of working with radiation. Table 9–1 taken from the BEIR-III[84] report gives the results of film badge monitoring on a sample of hospital personnel for 1975.

One can see from the table that most hospital-based radiation workers receive less additional irradiation due to their jobs than that associated with background variations within the United States.

Typically, the most heavily irradiated staff are those physicians performing brachytherapy (i.e., the insertion of radium tubes or applicators) and

TABLE 9–1.—DISTRIBUTION OF FILM-BADGE
DOSE RATE FOR HOSPITAL RADIATION
PERSONNEL IN 1975*†

FILM/BADGE DOSE (MREMS)	FRACTION OF PERSONNEL (%)	MEAN DOSE (MREMS)
Nondetectable	43.6	—
100	25.2	41
100– 250	12.6	159
250– 500	9.0	354
500– 750	3.45	618
750– 1,000	2.0	867
1,000– 2,000	2.53	1,391
2,000– 3,000	0.8	2,416
3,000– 4,000	0.25	3,391
4,000– 5,000	0.19	4,435
5,000– 6,000	0.08	5,457
6,000– 7,000	0.04	6,500
7,000– 8,000	0.03	7,443
8,000– 9,000	0	—
9,000–10,000	0	—
10,000–11,000	0	—
11,000–12,000	0	—
12,000–	0.13	128,425

*BEIR-III data. Used by permission.
†Data provided by Scientific Committee 45, NCRP, Washington, D.C.

84

angiography. In these areas, the physician is often faced with the moral choice of increasing his or her own radiation exposure (and risk) as a consequence of improving the efficacy of the patient procedure or in respect to the patient's safety. Nevertheless, it is instructive to note that even under these conditions, only 0.2% of all hospital workers exceeded the Maximum Permissible Dose guidelines promulgated by NCRP.

The concept of Maximum Permissible Dose must be clearly separated from the concept of Threshold Dose. The threshold concept is based on a nonstochastic evaluation of risk. That is to say, if an individual received a dose below the threshold, there is no risk of injury and the procedure is entirely safe (i.e., there is no risk of inducing cataracts by performing a skull series). The MPD concept is based on a judgment to which degree stochastic risk levels are acceptable (i.e., the chances are one in ten thousand that a worker receiving his thyroid MPD every year for forty years will die of a radiogenic thyroid carcinoma). The published MPDs should not therefore be thought of as safe levels but levels above which the radiation risks are considered to be unacceptable.

As has been previously discussed, low level radiation effects are often biologically and statistically indistinguishable from natural processes. The concept of a *de minimis* level of radiation is currently under discussion. The de minimus level is considered so low that it will be impossible to demonstrate any bioeffects from such a level. Therefore such exposures will not be included in individual or collective dose calculations. Proposals for the de minimus level range from 100 millirads/year (corresponding to background variations in the U.S.) to 0.1 millirads/year (corresponding to one brief air trip per year). The intention, at whatever level is finally accepted, is not to accept a dose below the de minimus dose as safe, but merely to accept it as a level below which the hazard cannot be measured.

The general philosophy followed by most radiation-using institutions is that of minimizing radiation dose (ALARA = as low as reasonably achievable). This concept includes radiation workers as well as the general public. The degree to which the policy of minimizing dose received by workers has been achieved in hospitals can be observed in Table 9–1. From this table we see that most hospital radiation workers received an occupational dose increment below natural background variations. Once occupational radiation exposures are reduced to this general level (de minimus?), it may be more beneficial to the employees if their employers spend "safety dollars" on reducing some of the nonradiation hazards at the work place.

In advising radiation workers, one must weigh the benefits of working with radiation against both radiation and nonradiation risks of such a job. As can be seen in Table 3–1, radiation work is among the safer occupations. Radiation protection standards for radiation workers are set at dose levels substantially below the level of nonstochastic risk and in a region of low stochastic risk. Since choice of an occupation is voluntary, a worker may choose to accept a greater statistical risk by working with radiation in exchange for the benefits (including avoiding the risks of other jobs) of such an occupation. Because the risk is small and confined to a small group, the dose limits for radiation workers are higher than for the general public.

There are a few myths about radiation workers that have persisted from the early years of the century. These include the provision of extra vacations and the "cultivation of an outdoor hobby" for radiation workers. While such advice is nothing more than common sense, a review of the early literature reveals that there was a concern for other factors, such as ozone and nitrous oxide emission from the generators of the day, electrical hazards from open wiring, as well as for the radiation hazards. Certainly, at the occupational radiation doses prevalent in the early days (several hundreds of rads per year), vacations permit time for biorepair of such acute injuries such as radiation dermatitis. At present, the risk of radiation exposure is stochastic. If we adopt the conservative linear, no threshold, no repair model of radiation risk, we must sadly conclude that extra vacation, if it does not reduce the total radiation dose received by an individual, is of no benefit in reducing radiation risk. Indeed, one could argue that a New York Hospital radiologist could conceivably increase his total radiation risk by taking a vacation in the mountains (an area of increased natural background radiation).

Another folk myth which has persisted in some institutions is the use of periodic blood counts as a means of radiation dose monitoring. Since an acute whole body dose of about 100 rads is required to produce a significant hematologic change, it is obvious that dose rates below a few rads per year cannot be monitored by such a technique. Hematologic studies as a means of radiologic dose monitoring are therefore only of value in the rare case of massive exposure. Chromosome analysis shows some promise as a biologic dosimetry system for doses in the tens of rads range. Such analysis is still in an experimental stage.

The occupational exposure of pregnant or possibly pregnant women is an area of special concern. The radiobiologic effects of fetal radiation exposure have been previously reviewed in this monograph. The general problem exists that while the mother is taking a voluntary risk in working with radiation, any resulting fetal exposure is involuntary on the part of the fetus. Female radiation workers are conscious of both the somatic and genetic risks to which their fetuses are exposed and often seek medical advice relative to such exposure.

The NCRP guideline is an occupational dose limit of 500 millirads received by the fetus during the entire pregnancy. The occupational and medical exposure of potentially pregnant women was reviewed by the NCRP[85] in 1977 and no modifications in the previous guidelines were promulgated at that time. In general, there is no problem in adhering to the 500 millirad/pregnancy fetal dose limit for medical radiation workers. As documented by individual film badge monitoring, most such workers receive less than 500 millirads per year, leading to a maximum fetal exposure below the guideline. The remaining percentage of medical radiation workers (mainly radionuclide handlers, fluoroscopists and their assistants) should be aware of their personal dose accumulation as monitored by their film badges. At dose rates below 150 millirads per month to the woman's skin (under the lead apron!) it is highly unlikely that the fetus could receive 500 millirads from the time of conception until pregnancy is established. The fraction of 1% of women occupationally exposed to dose rates exceeding 150 millirads per month should take special care to monitor their pregnancy status relative to their occupational exposure. Individual counseling is indicated for these few women. In all cases, the mother's tissues will absorb a significant fraction of the radiation, reducing the early fetal dose to about 50% of the maternal skin dose.

NONMEDICAL RADIATION WORKERS

There is a small but expanding category of nonmedical radiation workers. While employees assigned to nuclear reactors or nuclear fuel facilities come most quickly to mind, the category includes those laboratory scientists and technicians working with radionuclides or x-ray diffraction equipment, industrial radiographers, well loggers, shipyard workers, truck drivers, service technicians and members of other occupations. Generally these individuals know that they are radiation workers since they are issued film badges or other dose monitors. As in the case of medical workers, there is a wide variation in the actual exposure of individual industrial workers.

Both federal and state laws require that employers adequately inform their employees about the presence of ionizing radiation or radioactive materials; provide sufficient information to permit informed consent by the employees to their radiation work; and permit employee access to individual dose monitoring records. The ALARA concept, and its logical extension to minimizing collective dose to the employee population tend to keep exposure of the average worker well below the MPD. There are a few major caveats that apply to the industrial worker as well as those reviewed for the case of the medical work place: The employee should be aware of potential sources of irradiation and contamination, under both the normal working situation and under emergency conditions. The employee should be well aware of his or her actual radiation history; this includes the majority of workers whose radiation exposure is minimal as well as those few

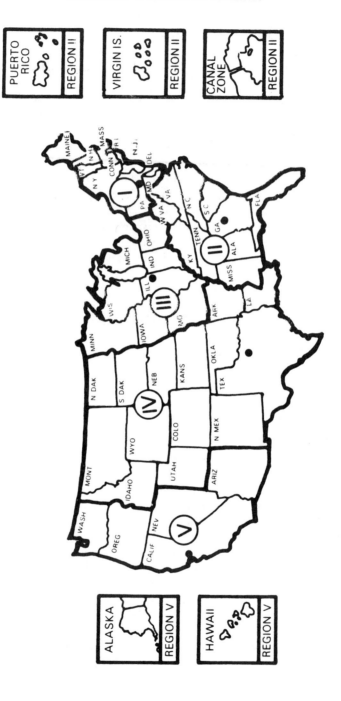

UNITED STATES NUCLEAR REGULATORY COMMISSION

A representative of the Nuclear Regulatory Commission can be contacted at the following addresses and telephone numbers. The Regional Office will accept collect telephone calls from employees who wish to register complaints or concerns about radiological working conditions or other matters regarding compliance with Commission rules and regulations.

Regional Offices

REGION	ADDRESS	TELEPHONE	
		DAYTIME	NIGHT AND HOLIDAYS
I	Region I, Office of Inspection and Enforcement, USNRC 631 Park Avenue King of Prussia, Pennsylvania 19406	215-337-1150	215-337-1150
II	Region II, Office of Inspection and Enforcement, USNRC 101 Marietta St., N.W., Suite 3100 Atlanta, Georgia 30303	404-221-4503	404-221-4503
III	Region III, Office of Inspection and Enforcement, USNRC 799 Roosevelt Road Glen Ellyn, Illinois 60137	312-858-2860	312-858-2860
IV	Region IV, Office of Inspection and Enforcement, USNRC 611 Ryan Plaza Drive, Suite 1000 Arlington, Texas 76012	817-334-2841	817-334-2841
V	Region V, Office of Inspection and Enforcement, USNRC 1990 N. California Boulevard, Suite 202, Walnut Creek Plaza Walnut Creek, California 94596	415-486-3141	415-486-3141

Fig 9–1.—NRC areas of geographic responsibility, their offices and phone numbers.

whose exposure approaches or exceeds the MPDs. The radiation and other risks of any job should be balanced against the needs of the worker and society.

Physicians dealing with transient radiation workers should be aware that their patients may be subject to irradiation at several different places of employment. These patients should be encouraged to keep an accurate record of their total occupational radiation exposure. The cumulative exposure of such individuals should not exceed the MPD guidelines.

RADIATION EMERGENCIES

While the authors think it unlikely that the reader will have to deal with a radiologic emergency, it is still worthwhile to review the principals of emergency management of radiation casualties. The key points are summarized in Table 9–2 and are discussed below:

TABLE 9–2.—RADIATION EMERGENCY PROCEDURE

---

1. In life threatening situations, the patient's other injuries take precedence over presumed radiation injuries.
2. If contamination is suspected, take infectious disease precautions (this will limit the spread of contamination).
3. It is highly unlikely that a radiation casualty presents a significant health threat to the emergency care team.
4. Hospitals accredited by JCAH have a radiation disaster plan and can supply specific assistance.

IN LIFE THREATENING SITUATIONS, THE PATIENT'S OTHER INJURIES TAKE PRECEDENCE OVER PRESUMED RADIATION INJURIES.—Most "radiation casualties" are seen in a context that also involves trauma (e.g., laboratory or vehicular accidents). As a guideline: Lifesaving emergency care should not be modified because of a radiation component of an accident.

IF CONTAMINATION IS SUSPECTED, TAKE INFECTIOUS DISEASE PRECAUTIONS (THIS WILL LIMIT THE SPREAD OF CONTAMINATION).—In emergency situations involving radioactive contamination, a major goal is minimizing the spread of the contamination. Such control can be accomplished by *imagining* the patient to be highly infectious. The same precautions and procedures which are used to control the spread of infectious disease (gloves, masks, control of ventilation, traffic and contaminated clothing) will serve to minimize the spread of radioactive contamination. Decontamination procedures should await expert help.

IT IS HIGHLY UNLIKELY THAT A RADIATION CASUALTY PRESENTS A SIGNIFICANT HEALTH THREAT TO THE EMERGENCY CARE TEAM.—Many radiation accidents involve only external irradiation of the victim. These patients represent neither a contamination nor an irradiation threat to their attendants. Most of the remaining cases involve contamination of the patient in small enough quantities of radionuclides so that these patients do not present an external radiation hazard to the staff provided that proper precautions are taken to minimize the spread of the patient's contamination. While not impossible, it is extremely unlikely that an accident victim be contaminated with large quantities of gamma emitting radionuclides. The very rare accidents of this type have occurred in facilities in which the first aid teams are well aware of unique special situations.

HOSPITALS ACCREDITED BY THE JOINT COMMISSION ON ACCREDITATION OF HOSPITALS (JCAH) HAVE A RADIATION DISASTER PLAN.—The JCAH requires that accredited hospitals have a radiologic emergency plan. These hospitals, and other facilities available to them, can act as a key resource in the management of radiation emergencies. It is therefore recommended that the nearest hospital be contacted as soon as possible after an accident.

The United States Nuclear Regulatory Commission is another source of emergency advice and help. The U.S. NRC maintains five regional centers that offer 24-hour per day response to emergencies involving radioactive materials. These offices, their areas of geographic responsibility, and their telephone numbers are shown in Figure 9–1. However, lifesaving medical care and contamination control should be accorded even higher priority than this kind of call for help.

Common sense predicts that the commonly seen "radiation emergencies" are likely to involve low levels of irradiation or contamination. While the authors regard all "radiation emergencies" as serious, one should not overreact to the radiation component of an accident relative to its other aspects.

10 / Public Health Aspects of Radiation

RADIATION, IN ALMOST ALL OF ITS FORMS, has been publicly perceived as one of the unique hazards of the last few decades. This perception appears to be related to the production of radiation and radioactive fallout by atomic weapons. The association of ionizing radiation with such weapons has been transferred in the public mind to associations with power reactors and medical imaging. Because of this chain of thinking, the general perception of radiation hazard is probably one hundred times greater than the real hazard. Such overestimates of radiation risk certainly encourage public and professional policies of minimizing exposure to radiation but may limit the beneficial uses of radiation.

The real hazards resulting from large doses of radiation have been known for at least eighty years. An appreciable number of early radiation workers were killed by inadvertent exposure to very high levels (thousands of roentgens) of ionizing radiation in the first decades of this century. Obituaries in the first volumes of most of the world's major radiologic journals report such deaths.[86] There is a monument to these radiation pioneers located in the St. Georg Hospital, Hamburg.[87] Professional awareness of the hazards of ionizing radiation led to the early publication of radiation protection advice[88] and to the formation of voluntary organizations such as the International Commission on Radiological Protection (ICRP).[7, 89]

There was a general awareness of the high dose radiation hazards by the 1920s. The exposure of radiologic workers has declined tremendously as a result of this awareness. At present, a dose sufficient to cause nonstochastic damage (~200 rads whole body) almost never occurs. Indeed, in a typical year there are only a few accidents that result in doses above 25 rads being received by anyone.

The scope and magnitude of radiation exposures can be seen in Table 10–1. In the United States, medical imaging exposes the population to a dose level that is approximately equal to the average natural background dose. Since this represents the major cause of man-made irradiation of the U.S. population and all radiation is presumed (for public health purposes) to be hazardous, a major public health effort is directed toward minimizing the unnecessary exposure of the population to imaging radiation.

PUBLIC HEALTH AGENCIES

The present collection of radiation protection organizations, rules, regulations and guidelines exists mainly for the purpose of minimizing the stochastic effects of radiation on the population. A second significant purpose of this network is that of the minimization of hazardous conditions that could lead to radiation accidents.

In this section, we will briefly review some key United States organizations with responsibility in radiologic health. There are many additional national and international organizations with similar responsibilities. The reader is encouraged to contact these organizations directly for more information.

NATIONAL CENTER FOR DEVICES AND RADIOLOGICAL HEALTH (NCDRH).— The NCDRH (5600 Fishers Lane, Rockville, MD 20857) is an agency of the federal government within the United States Public Health Service. The Center is responsible for the control of all medical devices as well as electronic products that produce radiation as an intended or by-product of their operation. It has been formed by combining the Bureau of Radiological Health (BRH) and the Bureau of Medical Devices (BMD). In the medical radiation area, the NCDRH has a key role in evaluating exposure of the population to diagnostic x-rays, ultrasound, nuclear medicine and radiation therapy. It works toward the minimization of unnecessary exposure both by regulatory control on the performance of x-ray equipment and by providing technical and biologic background information as well as advice to the medical profession and to the public. The NCDRH is, in addition, the major source of technical advice, technologic assistance and legislative recommendations used by state and local governments.

UNITED STATES NUCLEAR REGULATORY COMMISSION (U.S.NRC).—The U.S.NRC, Washington, D.C., 20555, is an independent agency of the federal government. The U.S.NRC is responsible for all radioactive materials derived from nuclear reactors. This responsibility therefore includes most of the radionuclides used for medical imaging. The U.S.NRC controls the safety of radionuclide imaging by means of extensive regulatory and licensing programs. Positive control of radionuclide usage by means of licensure is often delegated to state governments and to individual hospitals. The U.S.NRC maintains a staff of field inspectors whose duty is to verify safe usage of radioactive materials.

STATE AND LOCAL GOVERNMENTS.—All state governments and some larger municipal governments (i.e., New York City) have legal authority for the regulation of sources of radiation. This authority often includes the licensing of x-ray machines and radiologic technologists. NCDRH and NCRP

TABLE 10–1.—ANNUAL DOSE RATES FROM IMPORTANT SIGNIFICANT SOURCES OF RADIATION EXPOSURE IN THE UNITED STATES*

SOURCE	EXPOSED GROUP			AVERAGE DOSE RATE (MREMS/YR)	
	DESCRIPTION	NO. EXPOSED	BODY PORTION EXPOSED	EXPOSED GROUP	PRORATED OVER TOTAL POPULATION
Natural background					
Cosmic radiation	Total population	220×10^6	Whole body	28	28
Terrestrial radiation	Total population	220×10^6	Whole body	26	26
Internal sources	Total population	220×10^6	Gonads	28	28
			Bone marrow	24	24
Medical x-rays					
Medical diagnosis	Adult patients	105×10^6/yr	Bone marrow	103	77
Medical personnel	Occupational	195,000	Whole body	300–350†	0.3
Dental diagnosis	Adult patients	105×10^6/yr	Bone marrow	3	1.4
Dental personnel	Occupational	171,000	Whole body	50–125†	0.05
Radiopharmaceuticals					
Medical diagnosis	Patients	10×10^6 to 12×10^6/yr	Bone marrow	300	13.6
Medical personnel	Occupational	100,000	Whole body	260–350	0.1
Atmospheric weapons tests	Total population	220×10^6	Whole body	4–5	4–5
Nuclear industry					
Commercial nuclear power plants (effluent releases)	Population within 10 mi.	$<10 \times 10^6$	Whole body	<<10	<< 1
Commercial nuclear power plants (occupational)	Workers	67,000	Whole body	400‡	0.1
Industrial radiography (occupational)	Workers	11,250	Whole body	320	0.02
Fuel processing and fabrication (occupational)	Workers	11,250	Whole body	160	0.01
Handling byproduct materials (occupational)	Workers	3,500	Whole body	350	0.01
Federal contractors (occupational)	Workers	88,500	Whole body	250	0.1

Naval nuclear propulsion program (occupational)	Workers	36,000	Whole body	220	0.04
Research activities					
Particle accelerators (occupational)	Workers	10,000	Whole body	Unknown	<< 1
X-ray diffraction units (occupational)	Workers	10,000–20,000	Extremities and whole body	Unknown	<< 1
Electron microscopes (occupational)	Workers	4,400	Whole body	50–200	0.003
Neutron generators (occupational)	Workers	1,000–2,000	Whole body	Unknown	<< 1
Consumer products					
Building materials	Population in brick and masonry buildings	110×10^6	Whole body	7	3–4
Television receivers	Viewing populations	100×10^6¶	Gonads	0.2–1.5	0.5
Miscellaneous					
Airline travel (cosmic radiation)	Passengers	35×10^6¶	Whole body	3	0.5
	Crew members and flight attendants	40,000	Whole body	160	0.03
Airline transport of radioactive materials	Passengers	7×10^9‖	Whole body	0.3	0.01
	Crew members and flight attendants	40,000	Whole body	3	< 0.001

*BEIR III. Used by permission.

†Based on personnel dosimeter readings; because of relatively low energy of medical x-rays, actual whole body doses are probably less.

‡Average dose rate to the approximately 40,000 workers who received measurable exposures was 600–800 mrems/yr.

¶Total number of revenue passengers per year is 210×10‡; however, many of these are repeat airline travelers.

‖About one in every 30 airline flights includes the transportation of radioactive materials; assuming 210×10‡ passengers per year (total), approximately 7×10‡ would be on flights carrying radioactive materials.

"recommendations" may be enacted into regulations at these levels of government. In addition, NCDRH works with individual state governments for the surveys needed to establish data bases such as NEXT and contracts for the performance of surveys of certified x-ray equipment to determine compliance with the Federal Performance Standard. As noted above, NRC may delegate its licensing authority to individual states. The bulk of field radiation safety inspectors are employed at this level of government.

NATIONAL COUNCIL ON RADIATION PROTECTION AND MEASUREMENTS (NCRP).—The NCRP, 7910 Woodmont Ave., Washington, D.C., 20014, is a nonprofit corporation chartered by Congress. It is a free-standing organization of scientific experts in radiation protection. The NCRP, and its unincorporated predecessor, have published an extensive series of reports on radiation protection and related topics over the last fifty years. These reports are a compact source for the scientific background of most of the practical radiation protection effort in the United States. For example, Table 10–2 reproduces the table of Maximum Permissible Doses found in NCRP Report #39 entitled Basic Radiation Protection Criteria.[90]

PROFESSIONAL SOCIETIES.—Many of the professional societies have active programs in the area of minimizing unnecessary exposure to radiation.

TABLE 10–2.—NCRP DOSE LIMITING RECOMMENDATIONS*

Maximum permissible dose equivalent for occupational exposure	
Combined whole body occupational exposure	
Prospective annual limit	5 rems in any one year
Retrospective annual limit	10–15 rems in any one year
Long-term accumulation to age N years	$(N - 18) \times 5$ rems
Skin	15 rems in any one year
Hands	75 rems in any one year (25/qtr)
Forearms	30 rems in any one year (10/qtr)
Other organs, tissues and organ systems	15 rems in any one year (5/qtr)
Fertile women (with respect to fetus)	0.5 rem in gestation period
Dose limits for the public, or occasionally exposed individuals	
Individual or occasional	0.5 rem in any one year
Students	0.1 rem in any one year
Population dose limits	
Genetic	0.17 rem average per year
Somatic	0.17 rem average per year
Emergency dose limits—life saving	
Individual	100 rems
Hands and forearms	200 rems, additional (300 rems total)
Emergency dose limits—less urgent	
Individual	25 rems
Hands and forearms	100 rems, total
Family of radioactive patients	
Individual (under age 45)	0.5 rem in any one year
Individual (over age 45)	5 rems in any one year

    *Used by permission.

A small sample of the organizations whose efforts are most relevant to diagnostic radiology includes: the American College of Radiology (ACR), 20 North Wacker Drive, Chicago, Illinois, 60606; the American Association of Physicists in Medicine (AAPM), 335 East 45th St., New York, New York, 10017; and the Health Physics Society (HPS), 4720 Montgomery Lane, Suite 506, Bethesda, Maryland, 20014. These societies, and others, are excellent sources of relevant scientific information and practical advice. In particular, the ACR offers a set of patient handouts which very briefly review radiologic imaging procedures.

OTHERS.—The full list of organizations dealing with medical x-ray protection would exceed the size of this monograph. In general, the exposure of the population to diagnostic x-rays is well known. Positive steps are continuously taken, at many differing levels of responsibility, to minimize unnecessary exposure to this kind of radiation.

ENVIRONMENTAL PROTECTION

The radiologic community has the responsibility of minimizing the effects that their radiations have on the environment and on the general public. In this section, we will briefly consider the control of medical radiation as pollutants. There are two such pollutants that may pass out of the imme-

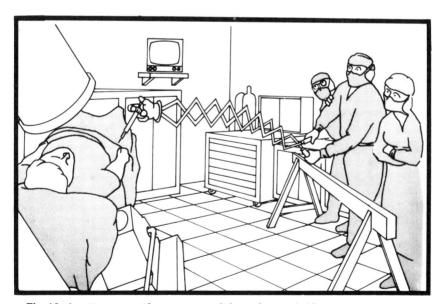

Fig 10–1.—Distance. The intensity of the radiation field is reduced by a factor of four every time the distance between the source and the observer is doubled.

diate control of the radiologist and into the environment. These are ionizing radiation and radioactive materials.

In each of these cases, one must consider both the amount of emitted radiation and the exposure potential of that radiation. For example, the emission of a large quantity of x-rays out the window of a fortieth floor office is not an exposure hazard unless there is another tall building across the street.

The general principles of radiation protection are well-known and readily applicable.[91] They are:

DISTANCE.—Doubling one's distance from a radiation source reduces the exposure rate by a factor of four. This is called the inverse square law (Fig 10–1).

TIME.—Minimizing one's time near an active radiation source minimizes exposure. Note that the average diagnostic x-ray machine produces x-rays for only a few minutes per day (Fig 10–2).

SHIELDING.—The use of sufficiently thick layers of any material can reduce exposure rates to as low a value as is desired. Lead is often used for

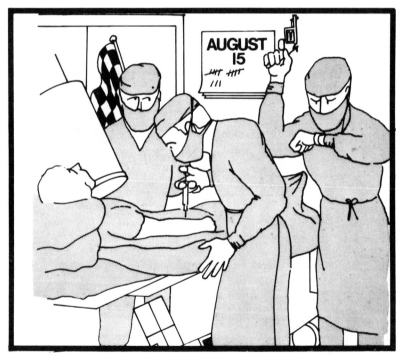

Fig 10–2.—Time. The shorter the time the x-ray beam is on, the fewer x-rays will be produced, and the less radiation received by the staff.

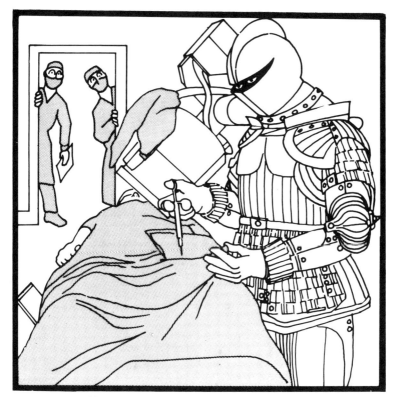

Fig 10–3.—Shielding. The radiation dose received by the operator can be reduced by the judicious use of shielding devices. Such protective devices include lead aprons, leaded thyroid collars, and eyeglasses containing high atomic number materials (with side shields) worn by the operator, as well as protective shields attached to either the ceiling or to the procedure table.

shielding diagnostic x-ray equipment because it is a very efficient attenuator of diagnostic x-ray photons (Fig 10–3).

These principles are used in combination to minimize the environmental hazards of radiation (Fig 10–4).

The presence of sources of external irradiation and radioactive materials is clearly indicated by means of "CAUTION" signs (Fig 10–5). These signs are intended to warn staff about potential hazards and to put them on alert so that proper precautions can be taken. Casual visitors to such posted areas should ask permanent staff for advice relative to appropriate radiation precautions. Qualified experts (i.e., physicists certified by the American Board of Radiology or the American Board of Health Physics) are often called upon to consult on the design of radiologic facilities. In addition to

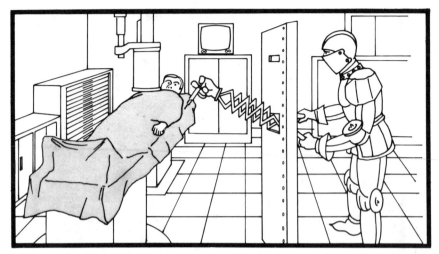

Fig 10–4.—Combining protective factors further reduces dose.

the "qualified experts," government inspectors, at several levels, regularly inspect radiation facilities to ensure compliance with safe practices.

Ionizing Radiation

It is possible to reduce the amount of radiation emitted into the environment by any single source to as low a value as is desired. It is pointless, however, to consider reducing the radiation dose received from such a source to levels much below those associated with natural background. Radiologic facilities are designed to legal standards which require that no individual in the facility's environs shall receive more than 500 millirads in a year. Most radiologic facilities maintain significantly more protection than the legal minimums. The BEIR Committee estimated that the average per capita dose from all miscellaneous causes (including the environment of radiologic facilities), is much less than 10 mrad per year. From this, one can infer that the environmental radiologic protection provided by most medical users is more than adequate.

Individuals working near radiologic facilities may be concerned about their personal exposure to radiation. While formal radiation surveys may indicate that there is no cause for alarm, it is the authors' opinion that short-term personnel monitoring (∼3 months) be provided to reassure the concerned person. Such monitoring should not be continued indefinitely.

Radioactive Materials

A prime concern in the handling of radioactive materials is that of avoiding the introduction of hazardous quantities into the environment. Many

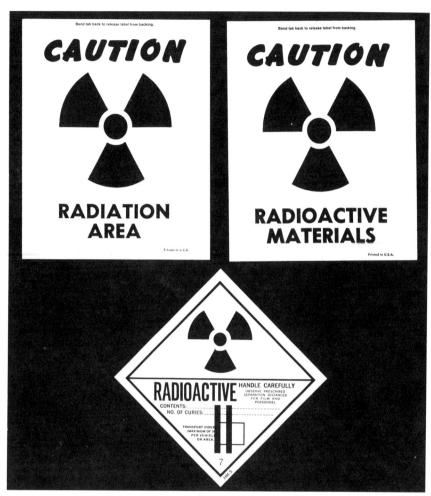

Fig 10–5.—Examples of common radiation caution signs. **A,** radiation area—possible external radiation hazard. **B,** radioactive materials—possble contamination hazard. (A radiation area sign is also used if there is an external irradiation possibility in the area.) **C,** radioactive—a label for shipping containers. This label is one of a series prescribed by the U.S. Department of Transportation for labelling hazardous materials in transit.

radiochemicals and radioactive wastes used in hospitals can be stored until the activity is eliminated by radioactive decay. In the case of ^{99m}Tc, a radionuclide used in large amounts in many hospitals, its six-hour half-life means that a sample stored for one week will have its activity reduced to 4 $\times 10^{-9}$ of its initial level. For a typical 10 milliCurie scanning dose the sample will have a decay rate of about 1 atom per second after one week's storage and a decay rate equal to 1 atom per year after less than two week's storage. Thus the storage of radioactive waste by hospitals or other users under controlled conditions will dramatically reduce their ultimate pollution potential.

Radionuclides, which cannot be stored until their activity becomes unmeasurable, are disposed of by dilution and dispersal (if gaseous or water soluble and in chemically nontoxic forms) or by transport to a licensed burial site. In the former case, the activity is so widely dispersed so that no individual can receive a hazardous dose. In the latter case (burial), the radioactive materials are confined until physical decay takes its course.

DOSE REDUCTION BY TECHNOLOGY

Technology offers potential means of reducing the patient dose resulting from a radiologic procedure. Even though a national survey of patient dose has not been performed since 1970, one can speculate that known improvements in equipment and procedures have contributed to dose reduction.

The cumulative effect of technologies on reduction of patient dose is difficult to access. As one example, a radiographic or fluorscopic system in use during the XES-70 study utilized between 25% and 33% of the image forming capacity of the x-ray beam. An efficient imaging system in the 1980s can utilize at least 50% of the beam. On this basis, one would expect a skin dose reduction relative to the XES-70 values.

Collimation of the x-ray beam to the region of interest is an example of an examination procedure that simultaneously minimizes the integral dose and improves image quality. The integral dose (total x-ray energy absorbed by the patient) is minimized by restricting the area of the x-ray beam. Image quality improves as the beam size is reduced as a consequence of a lesser production of scattered radiation by the smaller beam.

The reduction of the dose received by specific organs as a result of the utilization of improved x-ray beam collimation and gonadal shielding is difficult to assess in the absence of recent national survey data. Another factor that confuses the attempt to extrapolate XES-70 data in the 1980s is an increasing tendency toward tailoring the dose utilized in a particular examination to the requirements for image quality in that examination. Reduced physical image quality may or may not lead to a reduction in the diagnostic usefulness of an image. The tailoring of dose and image quality is therefore restricted to those examinations in which diagnostic accuracy is not compromised. The introduction of automation, including automatic collimation into diagnostic x-ray equipment, reduces integral dose. Other

TABLE 10–3.—ESTIMATED EXPOSURE REDUCTION (RATIOS OF VALUES REPORTED IN NEXT-80 AND XES-70)*

	RATIOS OF ENTRANCE EXPOSURE†	RATIOS OF MEAN MARROW DOSE‡
Chest, PA	0.9	0.8
Skull, LAT	0.9	0.6
Abdomen, AP	1.0	0.4
Cervical spine, AP	0.6	0.3
Thoracic spine, AP	0.6	0.2
Lumbosacral spine	0.7	0.4

*XES-70 is based upon a national sample drawn from the 1970 census. NEXT-80 is based upon surveys conducted in 17 states, with the origin of data biased toward Southern hospitals.

†XES-70 calculated skin exposures assume a standard man in place, thus backscatter is included. NEXT-80 ESE measurements are taken under low backscatter conditions. Therefore the ESE ratios have been corrected for this effect using BRH recalculations.[92]

‡Grossly different mathematical models were used to reduce the measured survey data into mean marrow dose in these two studies. These models were investigated by Rosenstein.[93] Data in this column is corrected for differences between the two models.

automation, the impact of the FDA equipment performance standards and the evolution of quality assurance programs in radiology departments, reduces dose by minimizing the need for repeat examinations.

This trend toward dose reduction can also be estimated by comparing the results of XES-70[14] with NEXT-80.[15] Table 4–1, previously shown, gave data drawn from those two surveys for a few representative radiographic projections. Rosenstein has applied corrections[92, 93] that bring both sets of survey data onto a more or less common base. These recalculations include accounting for different mathematical models used by XES-70 and NEXT for converting measured survey data into marrow doses. Additional corrections for scattered radiation were required on the entrance exposures because XES-70 assumed a standard patient was in place. The NEXT survey measurements were taken under low scatter conditions. Table 10–3 gives corrected ratios of the 1980 and 1970 exposures for both skin and marrow doses. Although this table suggests a reduction in skin dose and a substantial reduction in marrow dose, the nature of the required recalculations leads to a decrease in precision and thus obscures a truly quantitative comparison between the two studies. On balance, the authors estimate that the "dose" resulting from an x-ray examination performed in 1980 has been reduced by about 25% relative to the "dose" received in a similar examination in 1970. Wagner and Jennings[94] have recently reviewed sources of dose utilization inefficiency in radiologic diagnosis. It is their opinion that the per examination dose can be reduced by a factor of six to ten in the next decade. The authors of this monograph think that due to the intimate relationship between radiation dose and image quality and because of the relatively high utilization of the x-ray beam in 1980, such dramatic dose reductions are unlikely.

11 / Summary

WE HAVE TRIED TO SUMMARIZE the current state of knowledge concerning radiation-related risks in diagnostic procedures in radiology and nuclear medicine. We have seen that these risks are quite small especially when compared to other risks of life. Small, however, does not mean nonexistent. As in all other aspects of medicine, one must consider the risk to benefit ratio. Certainly, in those cases in which a definite disease state is expected or needs to be excluded, a study should be performed. However, when the patient's problem has not been carefully formulated by the clinician or if the clinician feels that the likelihood of a disease is vanishingly small, a diagnostic study is not indicated. Radiology is no substitute for clinical judgment, and such "fishing expeditions" are rarely productive. The clinician should resist the impulse to treat the patient's nerves (or his own!) with a diagnostic procedure.

We have also indicated our opinion concerning the optimal sequence of tests for a radiologic work-up of some common problems with a view toward the greatest yield for the smallest dose of radiation.

We hope that the material within this monograph will be of use to the practicing clinician, for it is his or her hands in which lies the greatest degree of control over the amount of radiation his or her patients receive.

Appendix A

RADIATION UNITS

Exposure. A measure of the radiation field.

$$1 \text{ Roentgen} = 2.58 \times 10^{-4} \text{ Coulombs per kilogram of air}$$

Dose. A measure of the energy absorbed per gram of matter.

$$1 \text{ Rad} = 100 \text{ ergs absorbed per gram of matter}$$
$$1 \text{ Rad} = 1,000 \text{ millirads}$$
$$1 \text{ Gray}^* \text{ (Gy)} = 1 \text{ joule absorbed per kilogram of matter}$$
$$(100 \text{ rads} = 1 \text{ Gray})$$

Dose Equivalent. A measure of the biologic effectiveness of a given quantity of radiation.

$$\text{Dose equivalent (rems)} = \text{Dose (rads)} \times \text{Quality Factor}$$
$$1 \text{ Severt}^* \text{ (Sv)} = 1 \text{ Gray} \times \text{Quality Factor}$$

(For diagnostic x-rays, an exposure of one roentgen will deliver a dose of about 1 rad and a dose equivalent of about 1 rem to muscle tissue.)

Activity. A measure of the number of nuclear transformations occurring in a sample of a radionuclide per unit time.

$$1 \text{ Curie (Ci)} = 3.7 \times 10^{10} \text{ transformations per second}$$
$$1 \text{ Becquerel}^* \text{ (Bq)} = 1 \text{ transformation per second} = 27 \text{ picoCuries.}$$

Half life. The time required for a sample of a radionuclide to decay to 50% of its initial activity.

$$A = Ao/2 \text{ in 1 half life}$$
$$A = Ao/4 \text{ in 2 half lives}$$
$$\text{Where } A = \text{present activity and Ao} = \text{initial activity}$$

---

*SI radiation units which are slowly replacing conventional units.

Appendix B

ESTIMATED MEAN EXPOSURE AT SKIN ENTRANCE (FREE-IN-AIR) FOR SELECTED RADIOGRAPHIC EXAMINATION BY TYPE OF EXAMINATION AND TYPE OF PROJECTION, UNITED STATES, 1970*

TYPE OF EXAMINATION	EXPOSURE AT SKIN ENTRANCE FOR EACH FILM (Milliroentgens)			
	A/P	P/A	LATERAL	OBLIQUE
Facial bones	320	440	190	—†
Sinuses	470	470	180	—
Skull	390	380	230	—
Cervical spine	270	—	170	200
Chest, radiographic	46	25	76	—
Ribs	350	280	—	—
Shoulder	190	—	—	—
Thoracic spine	670	—	1,460	—
Cholecystography	540	550	750	750
Cholangiogram	390	—	—	520
Lumbar spine	880	—	3,170	1,110
Small bowel series	—	670	—	—
Upper gastrointestinal series	610	540	1,110	750
Retrograde pyelogram	510	—	—	—
Abdomen (KUB)	580	410	—	—
Barium enema	760	770	4,010	1,350
Lumbosacral spine	980	—	3,540	1,610
Intravenous pyelogram	560	390	—	860
Pelvis	430	—	—	—
Hip	390	—	840	—
Pelvimetry	1,100	—	3,840	—
Cystography	310	—	—	—
Elbow	80	—	—	100
Hand and/or fingers	70	90	100	100
Wrist	80	110	80	140
Forearm	50	—	50	—
Foot and toes	120	—	120	120
Ankle	140	—	130	140
Leg	40	—	40	—
Knee	100	150	100	150
Femur	130	—	—	—

*Unpublished data from U.S. Public Health Service, 1970 X-Ray Exposure Study.
†Indicates insufficent data.

107

Appendix C

GLOSSARY

ABSOLUTE RISK. Expression of excess risk due to exposure as the arithmetic difference between the risk among those exposed and that obtained in the absence of exposure.

ABSORPTION. The process by which radiation imparts some or all of its energy to any material through which it passes.

ACTIVATION. The process of inducing radioactivity by irradiation. Diagnostic x-rays are incapable of causing activation.

ACTIVITY. The number of nuclear transformations occurring in a given quantity of material per unit of time.

ACUTE EXPOSURE. Radiation exposure of short duration.

ALARA. As low as reasonably achievable.

ANODE. The anode is the positive electrode within a tube toward which electrons are accelerated from the cathode. The kinetic energy possessed by the high-speed electrons is converted to heat and x-rays when the electrons strike the anode.

ARTIFICIAL RADIOACTIVITY. Man-made radioactivity produced by particle bombardment or electromagnetic irradiation, as opposed to natural radioactivity.

ATTENUATION. The process by which a beam of radiation is reduced in intensity when passing through some material. It is the combination of absorption and scattering processes and leads to a decrease in flux density of the beam when projected through matter.

BACKGROUND RADIATION. Radiation arising from radioactive material other than the one directly under consideration. Background radiation due to cosmic rays and natural radioactivity is always present. There may also be background radiation due to the presence of radioactive substances in other parts of the building, in the building material itself, etc.

BARRIERS, PROTECTIVE. Barriers of radiation-absorbing material, such as lead, concrete, and plaster, used to reduce radiation exposure.

BEAR COMMITTEE. Advisory Committee on the Biological Effects of Atomic Radiation (precursor of BEIR Committee).

BEIR COMMITTEE. Advisory Committee to the U.S. National Academy of Science on the Biological Effects of Ionizing Radiations.

BETA PARTICLE. Charged particle emitted from the nucleus of an atom with a mass and charge equal in magnitude to that of the electron.

BONE-SEEKER. Any compound or ion that migrates in the body preferentially into bone.

BRACHYTHERAPY (THERAPY AT SHORT DISTANCES). The treatment of disease with sealed radioactive sources placed near, or inserted directly into, the diseased area.

BRH. Bureau of Radiological Health (BRH). A former division of the United States Public Health Service responsible for radiologic health. Its functions have been incorporated into a newly-formed National Center for Devices and Radiological Health.

CARRIER. Nonradioactive or nonlabeled material of the same chemical composition as its corresponding radioactive or labeled counterpart; when mixed with the corresponding radioactive or labeled material, so as to form a chemically inseparable mixture, the carrier permits chemical (and some physical) manipulation of the mixture with less loss of label or radioactivity than would be possible in the use of undiluted label or radioactive material.

CHEMICAL SHIFT (NMR). A change in the resonant frequency for a given nucleus due to shielding of the nucleus from the external magnetic field as a result of the specific chemical environment. Thus, similar nuclear species bound to different chemical sites in a molecule will exhibit a shift in their resonant frequency, which can provide information regarding the chemical structure.

CHRONIC EXPOSURE. Radiation exposure of long duration because of fractionation or protraction.

COLLIMATOR, DIAPHRAGM. These terms are used somewhat interchangeably to refer to devices or mechanisms by which the x-ray beam is restricted in size.

CONTAMINATION, RADIOACTIVE. Deposition of radioactive material in any place where it is not desired, particularly where its presence may be harmful. The harm may be invalidating an experiment or a procedure, or in actually being a source of danger to personnel.

CONTROLLED AREA. A defined area in which the occupational exposure of personnel (to radiation) is under the supervision of the Radiation Protection Supervisor.

COSMIC RAYS. High-energy particulate and electromagnetic radiations which originate outside the earth's atmosphere.

CURIE (CI). Unit of activity $= 3.7 \times 10^{10}$ nuclear transformations per second.

DECAY, RADIOACTIVE. Disintegration of the nucleus of an unstable nuclide by spontaneous emission of charged particles, photons or both.

DE MINIMUS. A radiation level low enough to be considered legally trivial. A numerical de minimus value has not been established.

DIAGNOSTIC ACCURACY. An index of diagnostic efficiency, defined as the proportion of test results that are correct.

DIAGNOSTIC EFFICIENCY. A general term to denote the ability of a test to diagnose correctly.

DIAGNOSTIC YIELD. The proportion of test results that are positive.

DOSE. A general form denoting the quantity of radiation or energy absorbed. For special purposes it must be qualified appropriately. If unqualified, it refers to absorbed dose.

DOSE EQUIVALENT (DE). Quantity that expresses all kinds of radiation on a common scale for calculating the effective absorbed dose; defined as the product of the absorbed dose in rads and modifying factors; the unit of DE is the rem.

DOSE FRACTIONATION. A method of administering radiation in which relatively small doses are given daily or at longer intervals.

DOSE RATE. Absorbed dose delivered per unit time.

DOUBLING DOSE. The amount of radiation needed to double the natural incidence of a genetic or somatic anomaly.

EXPOSURE. A measure of the ionization produced in air by x- or gamma radiation.

EXTERNAL RADIATION. Radiation from a source outside the body—the radiation must penetrate the skin.

FILM BADGE. A pack of photographic film which measures radiation exposure for personnel monitoring. The badge may contain two or three films of differing sensitivity and filters to shield parts of the film from certain types of radiation.

FILTER (RADIOLOGY). Primary—a sheet of material, usually metal, placed in a beam of radiation to absorb the less penetrating components.

FLUOROSCOPY. Use of a fluorescent screen or image intensifier in rendering x-ray shadows visible.

FOCAL SPOT. That portion of the target of the x-ray tube which is struck by the electron beam.

FREE INDUCTION DECAY. The transient NMR signal picked up by the RF coil following switch off of the RF pulse excitation of the nuclear spin system.

GAMMA RAY. Short-wavelength electromagnetic radiation originating in the atomic nucleus.

GAUSS (G). The cgs units of magnetic induction field. 1 tesla = 10^4 gauss. (The earth's magnetic field is approximately 0.6 G at Washington, D.C.)

GENETICALLY SIGNIFICANT DOSE (GSD). The gonad dose from all sources of radiation exposure that, if received by every member of the population, would be expected to produce the same total genetic effect on the population as the sum of the individual doses actually received.

GONAD DOSE. The amount of radiation absorbed by the gonads resulting from any part of the body being exposed to x-rays.

GRAY (Gy). SI unit of absorbed dose of radiation = 1 J/kg = 100 rads.

GRID. A grid is a device similar to a grating whose purpose in roentgenography is to absorb scatter radiation which would impair the clarity of the image on the x-ray film.

HALF-LIFE, RADIOACTIVE. Time required for a radioactive substance to lose 50 percent of its activity by decay. Each radionuclide has a unique half-life.

HALF VALUE LAYER (HVL). The thickness of a specified substance which, when introduced into the path of a given beam of radiation, reduces the exposure rate by one-half.

HARDNESS. A relative specification of the quality or penetrating power of x-rays. In general, the shorter the wavelength the harder the radiation.

INCIDENCE. The rate of occurrence of a disease within a specified period; usually expressed in number of cases per million per year.

INTERLOCK. Several types of interlocks may be found in a radiology department, each serving to prevent the operation of a unit until a necessary safety precaution has been observed.

INTERNAL RADIATION. Radiation from a source within the body (as a result of deposition of radionuclides in body tissues).

IONIZING RADIATION. Any electromagnetic or particulate radiation capable of producing ions, directly or indirectly, in its passage through matter.

ISOTOPES. Nuclides having the same number of protons in their nuclei, and hence, the same atomic number; but differing in the number of neutrons, and therefore, in the mass number. Almost identical chemical properties exist between isotopes of a particular element. The term should not be used as a synonym for nuclide.

LATENT PERIOD. The period or state of seeming inactivity between the time of exposure of tissue to an injurious agent and response.

LINEAR ENERGY TRANSFER (LET). Average amount of energy lost per unit of particle track length in tissue. Low LET: radiation characteristic of electrons, x-rays, and gamma rays. High LET: radiation characteristic of protons and fast neutrons.

LINEAR HYPOTHESIS. The hypothesis that excess risk is proportional to dose.

LOCALIZATION, SELECTIVE. Accumulation of a particular nuclide to a significantly greater degree in certain cells or tissues.

MAGNETIC RESONANCE. The absorption (and emission) of microwaves or radio waves by electrons or nuclei respectively in the presence of a static magnetic field.

MAXIMUM PERMISSIBLE DOSE EQUIVALENT (MPD). The greatest dose equivalent that a person or specified tissue or organ shall be allowed to receive in a given period. Also see permissible dose.

MONITORING. Periodic or continuous determination of the amount of ionizing radiation or radioactive contamination present in an occupied region.

NATURAL RADIOACTIVITY. The property of radioactivity exhibited by more than fifty naturally-occurring radionuclides.

NONSTOCHASTIC. Describes effects whose severity is a function of dose; for these, a threshold may occur. Some nonstochastic somatic effects are cataract induction, nonmalignant damage to skin, hematologic deficiencies and impairment of fertility.

NUCLEAR MAGNETIC RESONANCE (NMR). The resonance response (absorption/emission) of a system of nuclei situated in a static magnetic field to an input of electromagnetic energy in which the width of the frequency response is narrow relative to the peak frequency. The frequency of the magnetic resonance coincides with the frequency of the Larmor precession of the nuclei in the magnetic field and is proportional to the strength of the field. The phenomenon is confined to nuclei having a magnetic moment (i.e., with non-zero spin). The resonance of such nuclei may be detected as they occur in ordinary bulk matter.

NUCLIDE. A species of atom characterized by the constitution of its nucleus, which is specified by the number of protons (Z), number of neutrons (N), and energy content or, alternatively, by the atomic number (Z), mass number ($A = N + Z$), and atomic mass. To be regarded as a distinct nuclide, an atom must be capable of existing for a measurable time.

PARAMAGNETISM. The property shown by many substances having unpaired spins thus possessing magnetic moments which tend to align themselves in a static magnetic field. This directional magnetization is not retained when the field is removed.

PERMISSIBLE DOSE. The dose of radiation that may be received by an individual within a specified period with expectation of no nonstochastic harmful result and low probability of a stochastic harmful result.

PERSON-REM (SYNONYM, MAN-REM). Unit of population exposure obtained by summing individual dose-equivalent values for all people in the population. Thus, the number of person-rems contributed by 1 person exposed to 100 rems is equal to that contributed by 100,000 people each exposed to 1 millirem.

PHANTOM. A volume of material approximating as closely as possible the density and effective atomic number of tissue. Ideally, a phantom should behave in respect to absorption of radiation in the same manner as tissue. Imaging phantoms are used to verify the proper performance of imaging systems prior to their use for imaging patients. Some materials commonly used in phantoms are water, Masonite, pressed wood and plastics.

PHOTON. A quantity of electromagnetic energy (E) whose value in joules is the product of its frequency (GK 37) in hertz and Planck constant (h). The equation is $E = h\nu$.

PIEZOELECTRIC. The property of inducing a mechanical deformation in a crystalline material by applying an electrical potential. Such materials will also produce a voltage when they are mechanically deformed.

POSITRON. Particle equal in mass to the electron and having an equal but positive charge.

PREVALENCE. The number of cases of a disease in existence at a given time per unit of population.

PROJECTION. A term for the position of a part of the patient with relation to the x-ray film.

QUALITY FACTOR (QF). The LET-dependent factor by which absorbed doses are multiplied to obtain (for radiation-protection purposes) a quantity that expresses the effectiveness of an absorbed dose on a common scale for all kinds of ionizing radiation.

QUANTUM. An observable quantity is said to be "quantized" when its magnitude is, in some or all of its range, restricted to a discrete set of values. If the magnitude of the quantity is always a multiple of a definite unit, then that unit is called the quantum (of the quantity). For example, the quantum of energy of electromagnetic radiation is the photon.

RAD. Radiation absorbed dose, or the specific energy absorbed at a particular point in a substance.

RADIATION. (1) The emission and propagation of energy through space or through a material medium in the form of waves; for instance, the emission and propagation of electromagnetic waves, or of sound and elastic waves. (2) The energy propagated through space or through a material medium as waves; for example, energy in the form of electromagnetic waves or of elastic waves (ultrasound). The term radiation or radiant energy, when unqualified, usually refers to electromagnetic radiation. Such radiation commonly is classified, according to frequency, as radiowaves, microwaves, infrared, visible (light), ultraviolet, x-ray and gamma ray. By extension, corpuscular emissions, such as alpha and beta radiation, or rays of mixed or unknown type, such as cosmic radiation.

RADIOACTIVITY. The property of certain nuclides of spontaneously emitting particles or gamma radiation or of emitting x-radiation following orbital electron capture or of undergoing spontaneous fission.

RADIOLOGIC METHOD. Techniques in radiography that are at the discretion of the physician, such as number of views, positioning, choice of contrast medium, length of exposure, patient preparation, etc.

RADIOPHARMACEUTICAL. A pharmaceutical compound that has been tagged with a radionuclide.

RADIORESISTANCE. Relative resistance of cells, tissues, organs or organisms to the injurious action of radiation. The term may also be applied to chemical compounds or to any substances.

RADIOSENSITIVITY. Relative susceptibility of cells, tissues, organs, organisms or any living substance to the injurious action of radiation. Radioresistance and radiosensitivity are currently used in a comparative sense, rather than in an absolute one.

RECOVERY RATE. The rate at which recovery takes place after radiation injury. Recovery may proceed at different rates for different tissues. Among tissues recovering at different rates, those having lower rates will ultimately suffer greater damage from a series of successive irradiations. This differential effect is considered in fractionated radiation therapy if neoplastic tissues have a lower recovery rate than surrounding normal structures.

RELATIVE BIOLOGIC EFFECTIVENESS (RBE). A factor used to compare the biologic effectiveness of absorbed radiation doses (i.e., rads) due to different types of ionizing radiation; more specifically, the experimentally determined ratio of an absorbed dose of a radiation in question to the absorbed dose of a reference radiation required to produce an identical biologic effect in a particular experimental organism or tissue. The ratio of rems to rads; if 1 rad of fast neutrons equaled in lethality 3.2 rads of kilovolt-peak (kVp) x-rays, the RBE of the fast neutrons would be 3.2.

RELATIVE RISK. Expression of risk due to exposure as the ratio of the risk among the exposed to that obtained in the absence of exposure.

REM. A special unit of dose equivalent. The dose equivalent in rems is numerically equal to the absorbed dose in rads multiplied by the quality factor, the distribution factor and any other necessary modifying factors.

RISK FACTORS. Characteristics of an individual, such as race, sex, age, other demographic variables, genetic variables or aspects of lifestyle which predispose the person to a particular disease.

ROENTGEN (R). Unit of exposure used in evaluating x- and gamma radiation. Defined as the quantity of x- or gamma radiation that will produce one electrostatic unit (esu) of charge, either negative or positive, in one cubic centimeter of air at standard temperature and pressure.

ROENTGEN RAYS. X-rays.

SCANNING (RADIONUCLIDE). The process by which the spatial distribution of a radionuclide within an organ or gland in the body is visualized.

SCREENING. Performance of a test in an individual with no relevant symptoms.

SECONDARY RADIATION. Radiation resulting from attenuation of other radiation in matter; may be either electromagnetic or particulate.

SENSITIVITY. The ability of a test to detect disease when it is present. Measured as the proportion of diseased individuals whose test results are positive.

SPATIAL RESOLUTION. The ability of a system to distinguish between two adjacent objects.

SPECIFICITY. The ability of a test to rule out disease when it is present. Measured as the proportion of normal individuals whose test results are negative.

SPONTANEOUS DECAY. The transformation of an atom of a nuclide into another form without outside intervention.

SPOT-FILM. A spot-film is an x-ray exposure, using a cassette or photofluorographic camera, made during the course of a fluoroscopic examination.

STOCHASTIC. Describes effects whose probability of occurrence in an exposed population (rather than severity in an affected individual) is a direct function of dose. These effects are commonly regarded as having no threshold; hereditary effects are regarded as being stochastic; some somatic effects, especially carcinogenesis, are regarded as being stochastic.

SURVEY, RADIOLOGIC. Evaluation of the radiation hazards incident to the production, use or existence of radioactive materials or other sources of radiation under specific conditions. Such evaluation customarily includes a physical survey of the disposition of materials and equipment, measurements or estimates of the levels of radiation that may be involved, and sufficient knowledge of processes using or affecting these materials to predict hazards resulting from expected or possible changes in materials or equipment.

SYMPTOMATIC. Any departure from the normal in function, appearance or sensation experienced by the patient and indicative of disease.

TARGET THEORY (synonym, hit theory). A theory explaining some biologic effects of radiation on the basis that ionization, occurring in a discrete volume (the target) within the cell, directly causes a lesion that later results in a physiologic response to the damage at that location. One, two or more "hits" (ionizing events within the target) may be necessary to elicit the response.

TELETHERAPY (therapy at long distance). The treatment of disease with x-rays of gamma radiation from a source located at a distance from the patient.

TEMPORAL RESOLUTION. The ability of a system to distinguish between two events that occur at nearly the same time.

TESLA (T). SI unit of magnetic induction: (1 tesla = 10^4 gauss).

THRESHOLD DOSE. The minimal absorbed dose that will produce a detectable degree of any given effect.

THRESHOLD HYPOTHESIS. The assumption that no radiation injury occurs below a specified dose.

UNSCEAR. United Nations Scientific Committee on the Effects of Atomic Radiation.

X-RAYS. Penetrating electromagnetic radiations whose wave lengths are shorter than those of visible light. They are usually produced by bombarding a metallic target with fast electrons in a high vacuum. In nuclear reactions, it is customary to refer to photons originating in the nucleus as gamma rays and those originating in the extranuclear part of the atom as x-rays. These rays are sometimes called roentgen rays after their discoverer, W. C. Roentgen.

REFERENCES

1. Hobbs B.: Adverse reactions to intravenous contrast agents in Ontario, 1975–1979, *J. Can. Assoc. Radiol.* 32:8, 1981.
2. Teplick S.K.: The biliary system, in Teplick S.K., Haskin M. (eds.): *Surgical Radiology.* Philadelphia, W.B. Saunders Company, 1981.
3. Seaman W.B., Wells J.: Complications of the barium enema, *Gastroenterology* 48:728, 1965.
4. Kaufman L., Crooks L.E. Margulis, A.R. (eds.): *Nuclear Magnetic Resonance Imaging in Medicine.* New York, Igaku-Shoin, 1981.
5. Pykett I.L.: NMR imaging in medicine, *Sci. Am.* 246(5):78, 1982.
6. International Commission on Radiological Protection: *Recommendation of the International Commission on Radiological Protection.* No. 26. Oxford, Pergamon Press, 1977.
7. NCRP: *Radiation Exposure from Consumer Products and Miscellaneous Sources,* Report No. 56. Washington, D.C., NCRP, 1977.
8. Cohen B.L., Lee I.S.: A catalog of risks, *Health Phys.* 36:707, 1979.
9. Slovic P.: Images of disaster; perception and acceptance of risks from nuclear power, *Proceedings of the NCRP* 1:34, 1980.
10. Upton A.C.: The biological effects of low-level ionizing radiation, *Sci. Am.* 246(2):41, 1982.
11. Fischhoff B., Slovic, P., Lichtenstein, S., Read, S., Combs, B.: How safe is safe enough? A psychometric study of attitudes towards technological risks and benefits, *Pol. Sci.* 9:127, 1978.
12. U.S. Department of Health, Education, and Welfare Public Health Service: *Population Exposure to X-rays, U.S. 1970.* Washington, D.C., H.E.W. Publication FDA 73–8047, 1973.
13. U.S. Department of Health, Education, and Welfare, Public Health Service: *Patient Exposure from Diagnostic X-Rays, An Analysis of 1972–1974 NEXT Data.* Washington, D.C., H.E.W. Publication FDA 77-8020, 1977.
14. U.S. Department of Health, Education, and Welfare, Public Health Service:

The Mean Active Bone Marrow Dose to the Adult Population of the United States from Diagnostic Radiology. Washington, D.C., H.E.W. Publication FDA 77-8013:8, 1977.

15. U.S. Department of Health, Education, and Welfare, Public Health Service: *Nationwide Evaluation of X-Ray Trends: Representative Sample Data 1980,* unpublished data.

16. Hammerstein G.R., Miller D.W., White D.R., Masterson M.E., Woodard H.W., Laughlin J.S.: Absorbed radiation dose in mammography, *Radiology* 130:485, 1979.

17. U.S. Department of Health, Education, and Welfare, Public Health Service: *The Selection of Patients for X-Ray Examinations.* Washington, D.C., H.E.W. Publication FDA 80-8104:24, 1980.

18. Balter S., Sones F.M., Jr., Brancato R.: Radiation exposure to the operator performing cardiac angiography with u-arm systems, *Circulation* 58:925, 1978.

19. Kruger R.A., Mistretta C.A., Houk T.L., et al.: Computerized fluoroscopy in real time for noninvasive visualization of the cardiovascular system, *Radiology* 130:49, 1979.

20. Ovitt T.W., Christenson P.C., Fisher H.D. et al.: Intravenous angiography using digital video subtraction, *AJR* 135:1141, 1980.

21. Proceedings of the AIUM Bio-Effects Committee, August, 1976: Statement on mammalian in vivo ultrasonic biological effects, *J.C.U.* 5:2, 1977.

22. Budinger T.F.: *Nuclear Magnetic Resonance Imaging in Medicine.* New York, Igaku-Shoin, 1981, chap 10.

23. U.S. Public Health Service Letter Announcement, Feb. 12, 1982.

24. National Radiological Protection Board: Magnetic resonance imaging, *Radiography* 47:563, 1981.

25. Webster E.W.: Estimates of cancer risks from low-level exposure to ionizing radiation: the BEIR report 1980, in *Biological Risks of Medical Irradiations,* AAPM Monograph No. 5:55. New York, American Institute of Physics. 1980.

26. Hall E.J.: *Radiobiology for the Radiologist.* New York, Harper and Row, 1978, p. 203.

27. Fabrikant J.I.: Estimation of risk of cancer induction in populations exposed to low level radiation, *Invest. Radiol.* 17:342–349, 1982.

28. Gofman J.W.: *Radiation and Human Health.* San Francisco, Sierra Club Books, 1981.

29. Pizzarello D.J., Witcofski R.L.: *Medical Radiation Biology.* Philadelphia, Lea & Febiger, 1982.

30. Report of the Committee on the Biological Effects of Ionizing Radiation (BEIR III): *The Effects on Population of Exposure to Low Levels of Ionizing Radiation.* Washington, D.C., National Academy Press, 1980.

31. Hall E.J.: *Radiobiology for the Radiologist.* New York, Harper and Row, 1978, p. 379.

32. Mettler F.A.: Updates on the UNSCEAR Report, AAPM Monograph No. 5:78. New York, American Institute of Physics, 1980.

33. Report of the United Nations Scientific Committee on the Effects of Atomic Radiation (UNSCEAR 77): *Sources and Effects of Ionizing Radiation.* New York, United Nations, 1977.

34. Seltser R., Starwell P.E.: The influence of occupational exposure to radiation on the mortality of American radiologists and other medical specialists, *Am. J. Epidemiol.* 85:2, 1965.

35. Matonoski G.M., et al: The current mortality rates of radiologists and other

physician specialists: deaths from all causes and from cancer, *Am. J. Epidemiol.* 101:188, 1975.

36. Jablon S., Miller R.W.: Army technologists 29-year follow-up for cause of death, *Radiology* 126:677, 1978.
37. Report of the Committee on the Biological Effects of Ionizing Radiation (BEIR-III): *The Effects on Population of Exposure to Low Levels of Ionizing Radiation.* Washington, D.C., National Academy Press, 1980, p. 501.
38. Merriam G.R., Focht E.F.: Clinical study of radiation cataracts and the relation to dose, *AJR* 77:759, 1957.
39. Report of the Committee on the Biological Effects of Ionizing Radiation (BEIR-III): *The Effects on Population of Exposure to Low Levels of Ionizing Radiation.* Washington, D.C., National Academy Press, 1980, p. 265.
40. Report of the United Nations Scientific Committee on the Effects of Atomic Radiation: *Sources and Effects of Ionizing Radiation.* New York, United Nations, 1977, p. 362.
41. Rugh R.: Why Radiobiology, *Radiology* 82:917, 1964.
42. Russell L.B.: Irradiation damage to the embryo, fetus, and neonate, in *Biological Risks of Medical Irradiations,* AAPM Monograph No. 5:33. New York, American Institute of Physics, 1980.
43. Gibson R.W., et al.: Leukemia in children exposed to multiple risk factors, *N. Engl. J. Med.* 279:906, 1968.
44. Stewart A., Kneale G.W.: Radiation dose effects in relation to obstetrical x-rays and childhood cancers, *Lancet* 1:1185, 1970.
45. Bithell J.R., Steward A.W.: Pre-natal irradiation and childhood malignancy: a review of British data from the Oxford survey, *Br. J. Cancer* 31:271, 1975.
46. Hoffman D.A., Felton R.P., Cyr W.H.: *Effects of Ionizing Radiation on the Developing Embryo and Fetus: A Review.* Washington, D.C., H.E.W. Publication, FDA 81–8170, 1981.
47. Report of the Committee on the Biological Effects of Ionizing Radiation (BEIR-III): *The Effects on Population of Exposure to Low Levels of Ionizing Radiation.* Washington, D.C., National Academy Press, 1980, p. 441.
48. Muller H.J.: Artificial transmutation of the gene, *Science* 66:84, 1927.
49. Taylor L.S.: *Radiation Protection Standards.* Cleveland: CRC Press, 1971, p. 35.
50. Schull W.J., Otake M., Neel J.V.: Genetic effects of the atomic bombs: a reappraisal, *Science* 213:1220, 1981.
51. Report of the Committee on the Biological Effects of Ionizing Radiation (BEIR-III): *The Effects on Population of Exposure to Low Levels of Ionizing Radiation.* Washington, D.C., National Academy Press, 1980, p. 82.
52. Report of the Committee on the Biological Effects of Ionizing Radiation (BEIR-III): *The Effects on Population of Exposure to Low Levels of Ionizing Radiation.* Washington, D.C., National Academy Press, 1980, p. 80.
53. U.S. Department of Health, Education, and Welfare, Public Health Service: *Symposium of Biological Effects and Characterizations of Ultrasound Sources.* Washington, D.C., H.E.W. Publication FDA 78–8048, 1978.
54. Bolsen B.: Question of risk still hovers over routine prenatal use of ultrasound, *J.A.M.A.* 247:2195–2197, 1982.
55. Meyer R.A.: Diagnostic Ultrasound: Hazardous or safe? *Appl. Radiol.* 11(5):71–74, 1982.
56. Kremkau F.W.: *Diagnostic Ultrasound, Physical Principles and Exercises.* New York, Grune and Stratton, 1980.

57. U.S. Department of Health, Education, and Welfare, Public Health Service: *The Selection of Patients for X-ray Examinations*. Washington, D.C., H.E.W. Publication FDA 80–8104:24, 1980.

58. U.S. Department of Health, Education, and Welfare, Public Health Service: *The Selection of Patients for X-ray Examinations: The Pelvimetry Examinations*. Washington, D.C.: H.H.S. Publication FDA 80–8128, 1980.

59. U.S. Department of Health, Education, and Welfare, Public Health Service: *Plain Skull Film Radiography in the Management of Head Trauma: An Overview*. Washington, D.C., H.H.S. Publication FDA 81–8172, 1981.

60. Whalen J.P.: Radiology of the abdomen: impact of new imaging methods, *AJR* 133:585,1979.

61. Burko H., Smith C.W., Kirchner S.G., Kirchner F.K.: Hypertension, in Eisenberg R.I., Amberg J.R. (eds.): *Critical Diagnostic Pathways in Radiology*. Philadelphia, J.B. Lippincott Co., 1981, pp. 199–211.

62. Lalli A.F.: *The Tailored Urogram*. Chicago, Year Book Medical Publishers, 1973, p. 61.

63. Sos T.A., et al.: Diagnosis of renovascular hypertension and evaluation of "surgical" curability, *Urol. Radiol.* 3:199–203, 1982.

64. Taylor K.J.W., Sullivan D.C., Wesson J.R.M., et al.: Ultrasound and gallium for the diagnosis of abdominal and pelvis abscess, *Gastrointest. Radiol.* 3:281–286, 1978.

65. Abrams H.L.: Observations on the manpower shortage in radiology, *Radiology* 96:671, 1970.

66. Hall F.M.: Overutilization of radiological examinations, *Radiology* 120:443, 1976.

67. Abrams H.L.: Sounding board: the overutilization of x-rays, *N. Engl. J. Med.* 300:1213, 1979.

68. Kelly K.M., et al.: Utilization efficacy of pelvimetry, *AJR* 125:66, 1975.

69. Campbell, J.A.: X-ray pelvimetry: useful procedure or medical nonsense, *J. Nat. Med. Assoc.* 68:514, 1976.

70. Roberts, F., Shopfuer, C.E.: Plain skull roentgenograms in children with head trauma, *AJR* 114:230, 1972.

71. Anderson R.E., Millikan C.H.: in Eisenberg R.I., Auberg J. (eds.): *Critical Diagnostic Pathways in Radiology*. Philadelphia, J.B. Lippincott Co., 1981, p. 312.

72. MacEwan D.W., et al.: Manitoba barium enema efficacy study, *Radiology* 126:39, 1978.

73. Shapiro S., Strax P., Venet L., Venet W.: Changes in 5-year breast cancer mortality in a breast screening program, in *Proceedings of the 7th National Cancer Conference*. Philadelphia, J.B. Lippincott Co., 1971.

74. A.C.R. Bulletin, November 1982.

75. Stitik F.P., Tockman M.S.: Radiographic screening in the early detection of lung cancer, *Radiol. Clin. North Am.* Vol. XVI, No. 3, Dec. 1978.

76. Heelan R.T., Melamed N., Flehinger B.J., Zaman M.B., Perchick W., Martini N.: The radiographic appearance of incidence non-small cell lung cancer in a general population of smokers. Presented at RSNA, December 1982. Paper in preparation.

77. Melamed M.R., Flehingher B.J., Zaman M.B., Heelan R.T., Hallerman F.T., Martini N.: Detection of true pathologic Stage I lung cancer in a screening program and the effect on survival, *Cancer* 47:1182, 1981.

78. A.C.R. Bulletin, October 1982.

79. Bydder G.M., Steiner R.E., et al.: Clinical NMR imaging of the brain: 140 cases, *AJR* 139:215–236, 1982.
80. Bolognese R.J., Corson S.L.: *Interruption of Pregnancy: A Total Patient Approach*. Baltimore, Williams and Wilkins Co., 1975.
81. NCRP: *Medical Radiation Exposure of Pregnant and Potentially Pregnant Women*, Report No. 54. Washington, D.C., NCRP, 1977.
82. U.S. Department of Health, Education, and Welfare, Public Health Service: *Procedures to Minimize Diagnostic X-Ray Exposure to the Human Embryo and Fetus*. Washington, D.C., H.H.S. Publication FDA 81-8178, 1981.
83. U.S. Department of Health, Education and Welfare, Public Health Service: *Gonad Doses and Genetically Significant Dose from Diagnostic Radiology*. Washington, D.C., H.E.W. Publication FDA 76–8034, 1976.
84. Report of the Committee on the Biological Effects of Ionizing Radiation (BEIR III): *The Effects on Population of Exposure to Low Levels of Ionizing Radiation*. Washington, D.C., National Academy Press, 1980, p. 52.
85. NCRP: *Review of NCRP Radiation Dose Limit for Embryo and Fetus in Occupationally Exposed Women*, Report No. 53. Washington D.C., NCRP, 1977.
86. Forssell G.: Heinrich Ernst Albers-Schoenberg: In Memoriam, *Acta Radiologica* 1:129, 1921.
87. Goerke H.: *75 Jahre Deutsche Roentgengesellshaft*. Stuttgart, Thieme, 1980, p. 74.
88. Desjardins A.V.: Protection against radiation, *Radiology* 1:221, 1923.
89. International Commission on Radiological Protection: *Protection Against Ionizing Radiation from External Sources Used in Medicine*, Annals of the ICRP 9(11). Oxford, Pergamon Press, 1982.
90. NCRP: *Basic Radiation Protection Criteria*, Report No. 39. Washington, D.C., NCRP, 1971, p. 52.
91. NCRP: *Radiation Protection for Medical and Allied Health Personnel*. Washington, D.C., NCRP,1976.
92. U.S. Public Health Service, unpublished data.
93. Rosenstein M.: Organ doses in diagnostic radiology. H.E.W. Publication FDA 76-8030, 1976.
94. Wagner R.F., Jennings R.J.: The bottom line in radiologic dose reduction, *Proceedings of the Society for Photographic Instrumentation Engineering* 206:60, 1979.

Index

121